The Neurosurgical Instrument Guide

D1434752

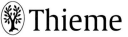
Thieme

The Neurosurgical Instrument Guide

Christopher S. Eddleman, MD, PhD
Neurosurgeon
Department of Neurological Surgery and Radiology
University of Texas Southwestern Medical School
Dallas, Texas

Thieme
New York · Stuttgart

Thieme Medical Publishers, Inc.
333 Seventh Ave.
New York, NY 10001

Executive Editor: Kay Conerly
Editorial Assistant: Daniel De Corral
Editorial Director, Clinical Reference: Michael Wachinger
Production Editor: Kenneth L. Chumbley
President: Brian D. Scanlan

Senior Vice President, International Marketing and Sales: Cornelia Schulze
Vice President, Finance and Accounts: Sarah Vanderbilt
International Production Director: Andreas Schabert
Compositor: Prairie Papers Inc.
Printer: Everbest Printing Co.

Library of Congress Cataloging-in-Publication Data: Available from the publisher upon request.

Important note: Medical knowledge is ever-changing. As new research and clinical experience broaden our knowledge, changes in treatment and drug therapy may be required. The authors and editors of the material herein have consulted sources believed to be reliable in their efforts to provide information that is complete and in accord with the standards accepted at the time of publication. However, in view of the possibility of human error by the authors, editors, or publisher of the work herein or changes in medical knowledge, neither the authors, editors, nor publisher, nor any other party who has been involved in the preparation of this work, warrants that the information contained herein is in every respect accurate or complete, and they are not responsible for any errors or omissions or for the results obtained from use of such information. Readers are encouraged to confirm the information contained herein with other sources. For example, readers are advised to check the product information sheet included in the package of each drug they plan to administer to be certain that the information contained in this publication is accurate and that changes have not been made in the recommended dose or in the contraindications for administration. This recommendation is of particular importance in connection with new or infrequently used drugs.

Some of the product names, patents, and registered designs referred to in this book are in fact registered trademarks or proprietary names even though specific reference to this fact is not always made in the text. Therefore, the appearance of a name without designation as proprietary is not to be construed as a representation by the publisher that it is in the public domain.

Printed in China

5 4 3 2 1

ISBN 978-1-60406-638-8

Contents

Foreword

Neurosurgical instrumentation is a complex mix of traditional tools shared by multiple surgical disciplines, coupled with instruments unique to neurosurgery dating back to the dawn of our specialty. This basic armamentarium is topped by a vast, confusing panorama of subspecialty tools whose individual structure and function remain opaque to most of us not initiated into the rites of that particular surgical cult. As confusing as this hodgepodge collection is to residents and fellows relatively new to neurosurgery, it is infinitely more difficult to navigate for our nursing staff and surgical tech partners on whom we and our operative procedures depend for rapid and reliable instrument identification and exchange.

Dr. Christopher Eddleman has done all of us involved in neurosurgery—surgeons, nurses, instrument technicians, etc.—a great favor by collating a common spectrum of neurosurgical instruments into a systematically presented text that not only visually identifies each tool, but concisely explains its function and common usage, details the multiple names by which it is often (and sometimes erroneously) called, and explains its usual place in the generic "sets" used by most operating suites. This innovative format facilitates the rapid identification of any instrument by sight, title, "nick-name," function, or normal association and is the essence of "user friendly."

Despite the fact that instrumentation is undeniably "faddish," out on the far borders of subspecialization, the core tools of our neurosurgical trade enjoy a remarkable longevity. That durability, added to Dr. Eddleman's compulsive exploration of even slight design modifications, and the thoughtful accessibility mentioned above, promise to make this unique, detailed guide a "must read" for young neurosurgeons and the gold standard reference for all neurosurgical operative services.

Duke S. Samson, MD
Lois C. A. and Darwin E. Smith
Distinguished Chair in Neurological Surgery
Kimberly-Clark Distinguished Chair
in Mobility Research
Professor and Chairman
Department of Neurological Surgery
University of Texas–Southwestern Medical School
Dallas, Texas

Preface

I vividly remember the days, both as a medical student and a junior neurosurgical resident, when the chief resident or attending neurosurgeon would ask for an instrument in the operating room, I thought they were speaking another language, especially when muffled behind their surgical masks. I can also remember surgical techs in training who had the very same look on their faces when the neurosurgeon's hand opened up for an instrument and they said, "ehofpiwefuiwdbcvpi." After some time, the neurosurgeons' voices became more understandable and the names of the instruments became clearer. However, some instruments were called three different names by three different people on three different occasions. How is one to learn these instruments and their names? Was it time and experience? Was there a neurosurgical instrument instructional text? Was there something I was missing in terms of instructional learning?

For neurosurgical residents, time and experience are how one learns the tools of the trade in the neurosurgical operating room. For surgical scrub nurses and techs, there are countless textbooks and guides that usually cover all surgical instrumentation (not just for neurosurgery) and with personalized instruction to boot. So yes, over time, and with a little experience, it is obviously possible to learn surgical instrumentation and all of their accompanying, quirky names. However, for neurosurgical instrumentation specifically, I thought there must be a better way or at least a way to facilitate the learning experience. Much to my dismay, there did not exist a book that was only neurosurgery centric. I thought that had to change and, ultimately, this instrument guide was what I envisioned.

The Guide's purpose is to take the basic neurosurgical operating room principles and instruments and give them some organization from a neurosurgical prospective. I also wanted to give a face to the names of the instruments called out in the operating room for the people who will not only be handing them out, but who will also be on the receiving end. Will this Guide allow one to walk into a neurosurgical operating room and know every instrument and its uses? Of course not. Does this Guide include every instrument in existence? Again, of course not. Does this Guide cover all of the subspecialty instrumentation for every minimally invasive spine, endonasal endoscopic, cerebral revascularization, and/or functional case? Definitely not! What it is intended to do, however, is to cover the basics—the neurosurgical instruments most often used day in and day out. Keep in mind, though, that some instruments can be used in many different procedures. As such, some instruments are included in more than one chapter. This only serves to reinforce the importance of that instrument and how it can be used in multiple areas.

The Guide begins with basic principles of the operating room, including arrangements, basic staffing, and equipment. Subsequently, basic instrument sets will be covered just to give the reader a feel for what could be included. Finally, each instrument is described from the perspective of a neurosurgeon. Each instrument page contains a photo of the instrument, an enlarged view of the working end(s), other alternative names, variations, and its general purpose during neurosurgical procedures.

What is not covered in this Guide is who makes them, where to get them, what they cost, and what they are made of. Several companies manufacture and/or distribute these instruments, and a consolidated list of the most popular companies is available at the end of this book.

Lastly, and most importantly, this Guide is meant as a learning tool, not a promotional one. Every institution has their pet set of instruments and/or companies which they prefer, and no one instrument is the "be all, end all." This guide is completely commercial-free and no company or manufacturer has been involved at any point in its construction. As such, any reference to any company or manufacturer that may appear herein is merely a byproduct of its production and is in no way meant as a promotion, as there are an infinite number of companies that have similar instruments available.

I hope this Neurosurgical Instrument Guide not only facilitates the basic knowledge of neurosurgical instrumentation, but also provides a lasting and progressively stronger comfort level in the neurosurgical operating room.

Acknowledgments

This Neurosurgical Instrument Guide has spent a long time milling around in my head. However, the living, breathing entity that you hold could not have been made possible without the contributions of many people. Significant time, energy, and tolerance have come from Lois Price, CST, Raechelle Robertson, RN, BSN, and Brad McGowan, MD. Of course, there are many others. Accordingly, and for fear of leaving someone unnamed, I will simply give those, and they know who they are, the grandest of gratitude. I am merely one member of a large team, for without any one of the other team members, this idea would still just be milling around in my head.

Chapter 1: The Operating Room

No guide to neurosurgical instrumentation would be complete without first discussing the operating room itself. While the instruments covered in this guide are used in the performance of neurosurgical procedures, the equipment in the operating room itself can also be thought of as instrumentation, involved in the workflow of the operation (**Fig. 1.1**). Knowledge of the operating room, its setup, and the basic equipment in the room *before* the patient rolls into the room will always improve the efficiency of the operating process.

Most operating rooms have a basic set of equipment and areas where the different personnel of the operating room staff complete their intended tasks before, during, and after every surgical procedure. That knowledge, along with awareness of the roles of each person in the operating room, further improves the workflow so that communication and tasks can be per-formed without delay, especially in times of potential crisis. In this chapter, we will review some of the basics regarding the operating room staff, general equipment in the operating room, and finally, basic operating room setups that are commonly used for neurosurgical procedures.

Operating Room Personnel

Most neurosurgical procedures that take place in the operating room, or "theatre" as it is called in the United Kingdom, Australia, and other countries, involve a team of people with defined roles, so that every need encountered during the procedure is met. Most operating room staff include a circulating nurse, a surgical technician or nurse, an anesthesia team (some with neuroanesthesia specialists) that may consist of an attending, fellow, CRNA, medical student, resident, and/or anesthesia technician, and finally, the surgical team itself, which may have several members, such as neurosurgery attending(s), residents, medical students, fellows, etc. Other accessory personnel who may be in attendance in the operating room include other medical students and residents not directly involved in the case, equipment or other industry representatives aiding in the use of specialized equipment, neurological monitoring technicians or staff, X-ray technicians, and pathology or laboratory staff awaiting tissue samples. The placement of each team member must be carefully considered before the procedure begins, so that no member hinders the operation or other workflow processes during the case.

Operating Room Setup

To ensure an efficient operating room, including all of the personnel mentioned above, the operating room must be set up so that all the team members and the equipment involved have specific places in the room. There are an infinite number of arrangements for the operating room, but a fundamental set of considerations must be addressed. Most operating rooms have supply rooms or closets that are located either in an adjacent room(s) or in cabinets within the operating room itself. These equipment areas should be accessible during the case without disturbing the surgeons and their team. The operating room table should also be set up to ensure that the transfer of surgical instruments between the surgeon and the surgical tech/nurse is comfortable and unhindered. The operating room setup should also place the anesthesiologists so that they have unfettered access to the patient's airway and vascular access lines. Further, the handedness of the surgeon must also be considered when the room is set up for a particular neurosurgical procedure to ensure that the exchange of surgical instruments can occur with precision and without obstruction. Lastly, and certainly important for the purposes of this guide, is the placement

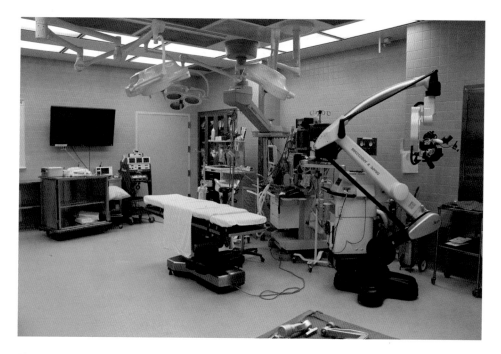

Fig. 1.1 Operating room.

and setup of the surgical instruments that will be accessed by the surgical scrub technician or nurse throughout the procedure. Other minor considerations that must also be addressed are the placement of the surgical microscope, the cauterization power supply and pedals, the surgical drill pedal, suction tubing, and similar equipment. In the next section, several basic operating room setups will be reviewed.

Basic Operating Room Arrangements

As stated above, the arrangement of the equipment and personnel in the operating room is very important for an efficient workflow during neurosurgical procedures. The diagrams below are very cursory and certainly do not cover every acceptable or conceivable variation. They are meant as suggestions and as a guide to teach how the operating room can be arranged to maximize efficiency. Both right- and left-handed setups are represented for general cranial, general spinal, and endonasal/transsphenoidal cases. More specific arrangements for specialized neurosurgical procedures are not covered but can be gleaned from the principles illustrated by the diagrams.

In all cases, the neurosurgeon's handedness is addressed by having the scrub nurse or technician immediately next to the surgeon's dominant hand, so passage of instruments proceeds without obstruction. However, as mentioned above, variations can and do exist. Two particular variations worth mentioning are prone and lateral decubitus positions. In prone cases, the scrub nurse or technician may be across the patient from the surgeon, so that instruments are passed directly to the neurosurgeon instead of from the side. Some feel this may allow better visual communication between the scrub nurse/technician and the neurosurgeon. In the lateral decubitus position, the position of the patient's face, and hence access to the airway, is fixed, giving the anesthesiologist limited positioning, even after extended ventilation tubing is put into place. The surgical scrub nurse or technician and the surgical assistant will more than likely be placed on the same side of the body. The important characteristic here is to always give the anesthesiologist a route to the airway such that crises can be averted. In the end, the arrangement is up to you or the facility that employs you. The important thing is to realize that there is a basis for where equipment and personnel are placed in the operating room (**Table 1.1**) (**Figs. 1.2, 1.3, 1.4, 1.5, 1.6, 1.7, 1.8** and **1.9**).

Table 1.1 Operating Room Setup Legend

A – Anesthesia
Ae – Anesthesia Equipment
C – Accessory Equipment
I – Surgical Instruments
M – Microscope
S – Neurosurgeon
s – Assistant Neurosurgeon
Sn – Scrub Nurse or Tech

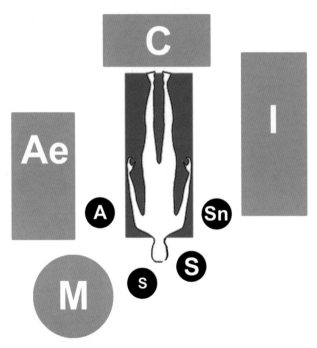

Fig. 1.2 General right-handed surgeon supine or posterior fossa craniotomy setup (cranial approach).

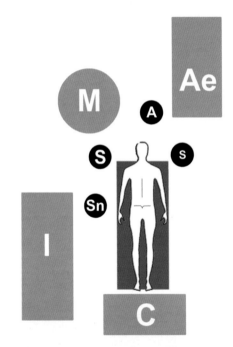

Fig. 1.3 General right-handed surgeon posterior fossa craniotomy setup (caudal approach).

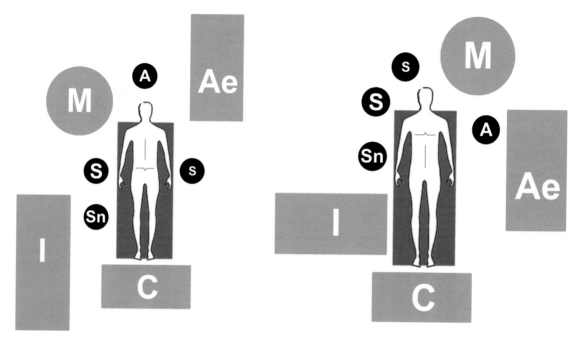

Fig. 1.4 General right-handed surgeon spine procedure setup.

Fig. 1.5 General right-handed surgeon endonasal/transsphenoidal setup.

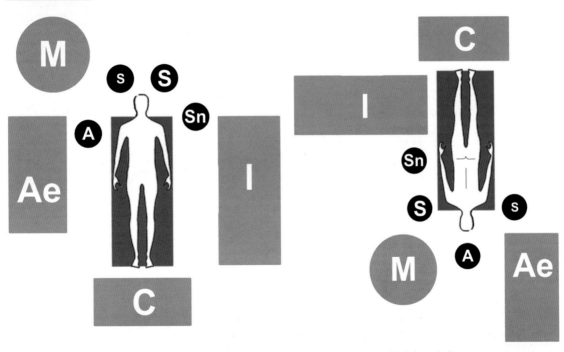

Fig. 1.6 General left-handed surgeon supine or posterior fossa craniotomy setup (cranial approach).

Fig. 1.7 General left-handed surgeon posterior fossa craniotomy setup (caudal approach).

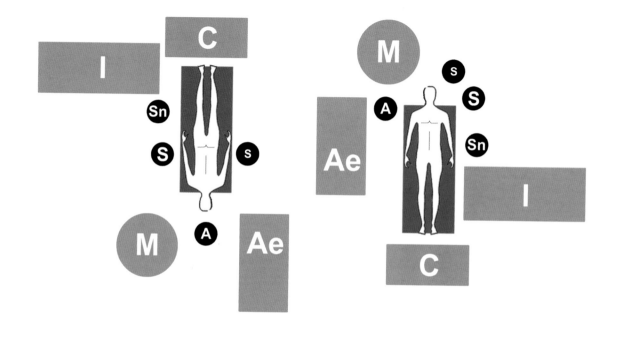

Fig.1.8 General left-handed surgeon spine procedure setup.

Fig.1.9 General left-handed surgeon endonasal/transsphenoidal setup.

Chapter 2: Operating Room Equipment

While neurosurgical instruments are the main focus in this guide, there is certainly a myriad of equipment in the operating room that should also be considered essential pieces of neurosurgical equipment knowledge.

One of the most important pieces of equipment is the operating room table. Several different kinds of operating room tables are used, and the choice is often dependent on the type of neurosurgical procedure involved. The standard operating room table (**Fig. 2.1**) has many sections that allow a wide range of patient positions. Most people should be familiar with the tables' controls and the different positions that these tables make possible. Most tables will also rotate to allow "airplaning" (lateral turning) the patient in either direction, so that more precise positioning can be obtained before and during most neurosurgical procedures. Most neuro-

surgical procedures involving patients in the supine, sitting, and lateral positions can utilize a similar table. When a head holder is needed for supine patients, the most common are the Mayfield-Keys (**Fig. 2.2**) or the "horseshoe" (**Fig. 2.3**) head holders. For those patients undergoing a prone position procedure involving the head or cervical spine, this same table can be used with chest rolls and a stabilizing head holder, most commonly the Mayfield-Keys head holder. Spine procedures involving opening the disc spaces utilizing this general operating room table can utilize a Wilson frame added to the top of this operating room table. The Wilson frame arches the back and facilitates access to the disc spaces. For more extensive spine procedures, a different type of table is often used, which has an open construction, so the table does not compress the patient's abdomen. A Jackson table, one of

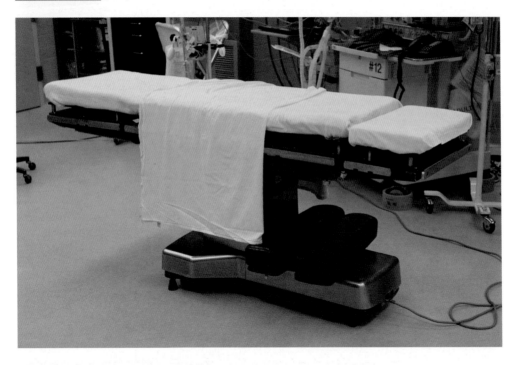

Fig. 2.1 Basic operating room table.

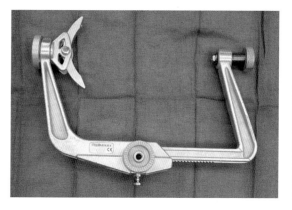

Fig. 2.2 Mayfield-Keys headholder.

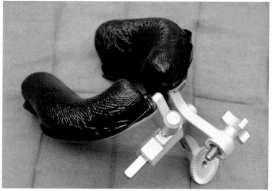

Fig. 2.3 Horseshoe.

many of this type, has adjustable padding attachments on the sides to support the bony aspects of the pelvis while also padding the upper chest and providing flat panels for the knees. These tables are highly diverse in terms of what attachments can be added as well as how the table can be positioned. Most can be rotated, raised, or put in Trendelenburg positions. Other types of attachments serve the purposes of positioning, padding, and providing points for securing other pieces of equipment, such as arms or retractors.

Of particular note, many different attachments to the operating room table or head holder are retraction systems. Several of them are used throughout the world, but the three most common are the Leyla-Yasargil, Budde Halo, and the Greenberg retraction systems. The Leyla-Yasargil retraction system is connected to the Leyla bar, which is stabilized to the operating room table. A connector box affixed at the end of the bar serves as the centerpiece to which all of the retraction arms are connected. The Budde Halo and the Greenberg retraction systems can be connected to the operating room table or to the head holder. These retraction systems afford the neurosurgeon hands-free retraction. Further, the Budde Halo can provide the neurosurgeon an arm rest while working.

Another important piece of equipment in the operating room is the cart containing the power sources for the electrocautery devices, electric drills, and other equipment that requires a power source (**Fig. 2.4**). It is important to know the placement of such equipment so that the cables needed to connect to them can be placed properly in the operative field. While the operating room staff will normally perform this task, setting up the operating room in the

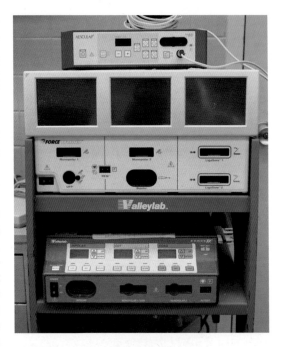

Fig. 2.4   Accessory equipment.

middle of the night might require you to do this task, making it very important to sustain an efficient workflow.

The overhead operating room lights are often overlooked pieces of equipment that are highly important to performance of neurosurgical procedures. It is important to know the range of mobility of the lights and to have them set up at the beginning of the case. This ensures that you are not fumbling around at the beginning to position the lights with a sterile field in the way.

Lastly, as shown in the diagrams in Chapter 1, the microscope is an important piece of equipment that one should become very familiar with before the start of a case. It is very important to place the microscope so it does not impede the symphony of neurosurgical instrument exchanges. Further, it is of paramount importance to place the observer scopes in positions where the assistant does not impede the surgical technician when exchanging instruments.

Many more pieces of equipment are found in the operating room, and one should be familiar with them before beginning a neurosurgical case. If you are not sure of something, do not be afraid to ask. Once this knowledge is set and understood, then the process of learning the neurosurgical instruments can begin.

Chapter 3: Basic Neurosurgical Trays

Despite the vast array of neurosurgical procedures that are performed from head to toe, most neurosurgical procedures can be done with the use of basic instrument sets, which may be somewhat tailored to the procedure. The three most common neurosurgical instrument sets are cranial, spine, and transsphenoidal. At some institutions, a trauma instrument tray may be available, but often the cranial set can be used in its place. Academic institutions, at least in the United States, will often have a litany of more specific instrument trays available for more specific procedures, e.g., functional, peripheral nerve, CSF shunts, neurovascular, carotid, cerebral revascularization, minimally invasive, complex spine, and others.

The following lists of basic neurosurgical instrument sets are only meant as a starting point and are not meant to define what these sets should be, but to illustrate what they could be. Every conceivable instrument that could be placed in a "basic" set is not listed here. Images and descriptions of these instruments are contained throughout the rest of this guide. The numbers of instruments to include frequently depend on the allotted and available budget. Normally, each set can contain one of each variety of scissors, curettes, dissectors, and rongeurs, while clamps, forceps, suction tips, retractors, and elevators are usually present in multiple numbers of the same type. Several companies and worldwide distributors offer start-up sets that are able to fit most budgets. The World Federation of Neurosurgeons also has basic neurosurgical instrument sets available to parts of the world that lack sufficient supply and capital.

Basic Cranial or Trauma Instrument Set

Scissors

Adson ganglion 6¼"
Malis neurological 7" curved
Mayo 6¾" curved beveled
Metzenbaum 7" curved
Potts-DeMartel 7¼" 45°
Shark Edge Mayo-Stille 6¾" straight

Needle holders

Mayo-Hegar 6" heavy
Ryder 6" X-Del
Ryder 7" X-Del

Clamps

Allis 6" straight
Foerster sponge stick 9½" straight
Halstead mosquito 5" straight
Kelly 5½" curved
Kocher 6" straight
Rochester-Pean 7¼" Curved

Dissectors/hooks

Dandy nerve hook 9" straight
Frazier dura hook 5¼"
Joseph double hook 6½"
Penfield 1–4
Woodson dural separator 7"

Elevators

Langenbeck 7½" 16 mm
Quervain 7¾" 6 mm

Knife handles

#3 with ruler
#7 without ruler

Forceps

Adson 4¾" with teeth
Gerald 7" with teeth
Gruenwald Bayo 8"
Tissue 5¾" straight with teeth
Yasargil rumor 8¾"

Suction tips

    Poppen 5½" angled 7 Fr, 9–12 Fr (Frazier)

    Dental irrigator

Miscellaneous

    Army-Navy retractor

    Backhaus towel clips 5¼", 3½"

    Beyer rongeur 7" Curved double action 4.5×19 mm (Ruskin)

    Cushing retractor 8⅜"

    Fish hooks with Songer cables

    Freiburg spatula 8" mall flat 7/8, 10/11, 13/14, 16/17 mm

    Gelpi retractor 7¼"

Hemoclip applier traditional 8" curved, medium

Hemoclip applier traditional 6" curved, small

Kerrison rongeur 2–3 mm

Leksell-Stille rongeur 9½" angled double-action 7.5×22 mm

Mastoid retractor 7⅞" 4×4 Prong sharp

Raney appliers

Screwdriver with blades

Spinal fusion curette 6¾" angled

Stille rongeur 9¼" double action (duckbill)

Volkmann bone curette 6¾" 3.6 mm

Weitlaner retractor 6½" blunt 3×4

Basic Spinal Instrument Set

Scissors

Adson ganglion 6¼" straight
Angular wire 4¾"
Mayo 6¾" curved
Mayo 6¾" straight
Metzenbaum 5" curved
Metzenbaum 7" curved
Potts 7¼", angled 45°

Needle holders

Crile Wood 6"
Mayo-Hegar 6"
Mayo-Hegar 8" heavy

Clamps

Adson 7½" straight
Allis 6"
Crile 5¾" curved
Foerster sponge stick 9½" straight
Halstead mosquito 5" straight
Hemoclip applier traditional 8" curved,
    medium
Lewin bone 7"
Mayo-Pean 7" curved
Ochsner 6¼" straight
Right angle

Forceps

Adson 4¾" with teeth
Cushing with teeth
Gerald 7" with teeth
Gruenwald Bayo 8½" without teeth
Smooth pickup

Knife handles

#3 with ruler
#7 without ruler

Dissectors

Dandy nerve hook 9" straight
Penfield 1,2,3,4
Woodson dural separator 7"

Suction

Frazier 7Fr, 9Fr, 12Fr

Curette

Spinal fusion 9" straight (multiple sizes)
Spinal fusion 9" angled (multiple sizes)

Retractor

Army-Navy
Collis-Taylor 7¼" 76 mm
Collis-Taylor 7¼" 64 mm
Gelpi 7½"
Love nerve root 8¼", angled 90°
Weitlaner 6½" 3×4 sharp

Miscellaneous

Backhaus towel clip 5¼"
Backhaus towel clip 3½"
Cobb spinal elevator ⅜",½",¾"
Langenbeck periosteal elevators
Leksell rongeur 9" wide 8 mm
Leksell rongeur 8½" full curved
   8×16 mm
Dental irrigators

Basic Transsphenoidal Instrument Set

Retractors

Army-Navy
Cottle speculum short 9×30 mm, 5¾" 2 mm, 10×70 mm
Hardy bivalve speculum 2¾", 3½", 3⅛"
Killian nasal speculum 5" extra-large 85×8.5 mm
Rhoton transsphenoidal speculum small
Weitlaner 5½" 3×4 blunt

Clamps

Allis 6"
Backhaus towel clips 3, 5½"
Halstead mosquito 5" straight
Kelly 5½" curved
Kocher Ochsner 7¼" straight
Micro Halstead 5" curved

Needle holders

Jacobson Bayo 6⅜"

Mayo Hegar 6", 7" heavy
Webster 5¾"

Scissors

Adson ganglion 6½" straight
Becker septum 7" straight
Knapp iris
Knight nasal
Mayo 6¾" curved, straight, beveled
Metzenbaum 7" curved
Micro cut up-angled, straight
Nasal sinus right, left, 8¾" straight

Forceps

Adson with teeth
Brown-Adson 4¾"
Gruenwald Bayo 8" without teeth
Jansen-Middleton 7" angled down 4×11 mm, 8¼" angled down
Sinus cup (Takahashi pituitary Oldberg)
Takahashi 6¾" straight 3 mm, 6¾" 4 mm

Knives and handles

- #7 knife handles
- #3 knife handle with ruler
- Sickle knife 7½" straight sharp tip adult
- Freer knife 6" round
- Ballenger swivel knife 7½" straight 4 mm

Rongeurs

- Kerrison 7" 40°, 45°, 90° thin foot 1–3 mm, 2–3 mm
- Decker micro 6" 2×6 mm
- Beyer rongeur 7" curved double action 4.5×19 mm (Ruskin)
- Ostrum Antrum straight
- Blakesley Wilde Rhinoforce 45°
- Yasargil pituitary 7½" straight 3.5 mm
- Oldberg pituitary 7" straight 7 mm

Miscellaneous

- Cottle mallet 8" 30 mm
- Poppen (Frazier) suction 5–11 Fr
- Dental irrigator
- Foerster sponge stick 9¾" straight
- Converse osteotome 7" straight 4 mm, 6 mm, 8 mm
- Cottle elevator
- Boles elevator 7" blunt
- Fomon retractor ball
- Joseph skin hook 6½" single, double prong
- Freer elevator 7½" 4.5 mm
- Gorney septum elevator suction
- Maxillary ostium seeker 7½"

Chapter 4: Basic Neurological Instrumentation

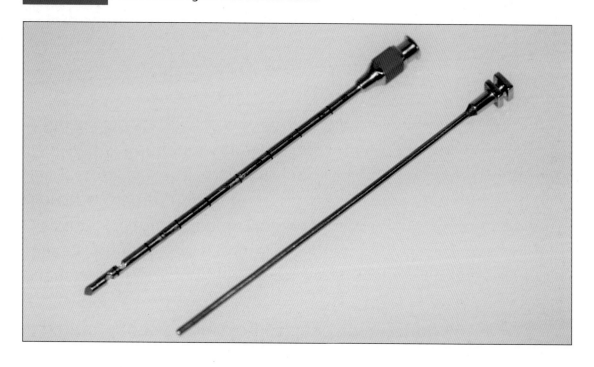

Brain Needle

Alternative Name: None

Category: General

Purposes: Used to establish a trajectory in the brain toward a particular target, e.g., ventricle for CSF drainage or mass for biopsy. Smooth end and shaft allow less traumatic trajectory through brain tissue. Stylet can be removed to confirm position or can be used with navigation systems for stereotactic guidance.

Varieties: Lengths of shaft.

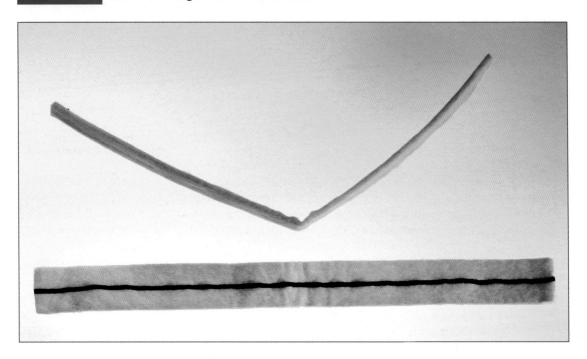

Cotton Patty

Alternative Names: Patty, strip, called out by the measurement of the patty (e.g., half by half), cotton strip or patty

Category: General

Purposes: Multipurpose cotton patties, more commonly used in hemostasis maneuvers involving Gelfoam, Surgicel, or other hemostatic agents. The patty is placed over the agent and the suction draws either blood or fluid, facilitating coagulation. Can be used to apply bone wax atraumatically. Also used as either a wick to draw fluid away or as a protection barrier over vital structures. Many other uses exist. Has a radiopaque strip down the middle.

Varieties: Square and rectangular shapes. Multiple sizes.

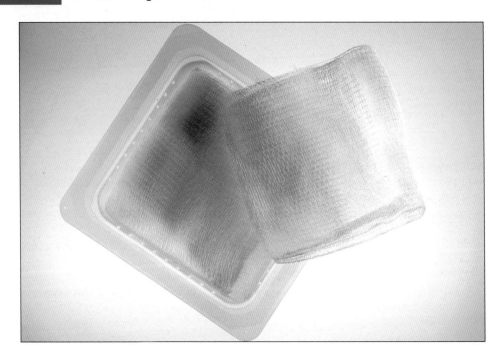

Cotton Sponge

Alternative Names: Ray-tec, sponge, 4×4

Category: General

Purposes: Cotton sheets serving a multitude of purposes, e.g., cleaning, hemostasis, wicking, holding tissue, placement under skin flaps, etc. Filament in sponge allows X-ray detection.

Varieties: Various sizes.

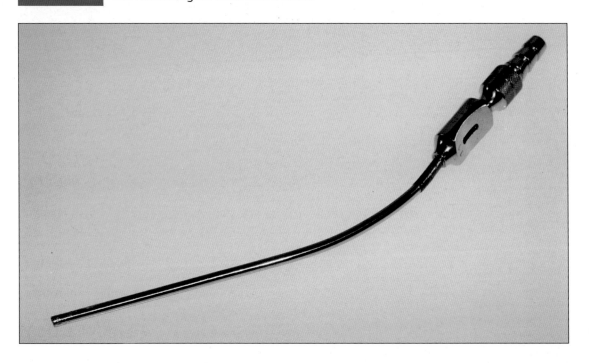

Frazier Suction

Alternative Name: Poppen suction

Category: General

Purposes: Used for suction of fluids in confined spaces. Thumb hole allows on-and-off style of suction. Also used as a retractor, protection device, and blunt dissection tool, when removing tumor or brain parenchyma.

Varieties: Straight or angled. Various diameters of tips.

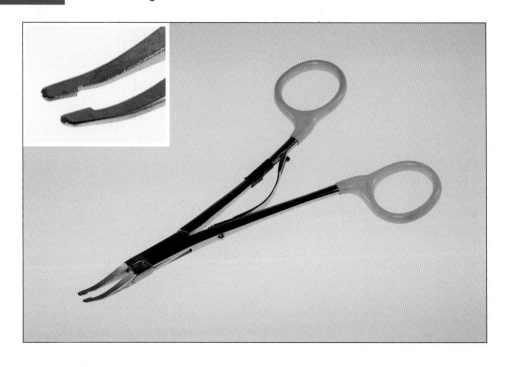

Hemoclip Applier

Alternative Names: Ligaclip applier, vascular clip applier, vessel clip applier

Category: General

Purposes: Used for applying small metal clips for occlusion of vessels. Multiple sizes of clips are available for a diverse range of vessel sizes.

Varieties: Accommodation of various sized clips. Variable lengths.

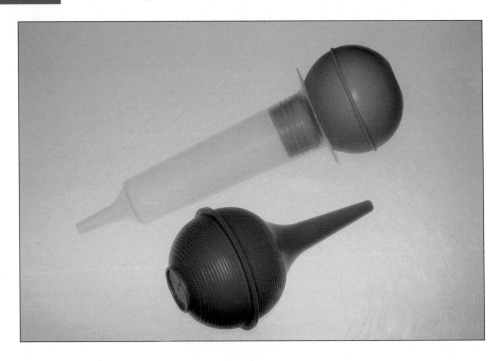

Irrigator

Alternative Names: Asepto, Asepto syringe, bulb syringe, water, big irrigation, flush

Category: General

Purposes: Refillable bulb syringes used for directed irrigation of the surgical site.

Varieties: Multiple sizes and shapes of syringes.

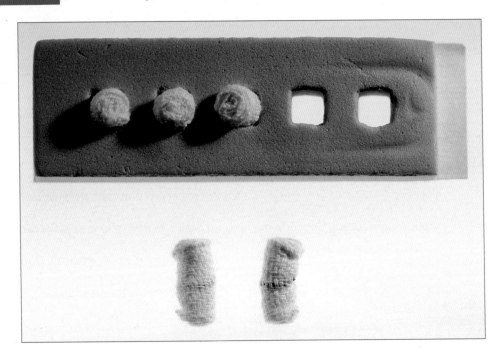

Kittner

Alternative Name: Peanut

Category: General

Purposes: Small rolled-up gauze usually held by a Kelly, Crile, or mosquito clamp and used to dissect tissue bluntly or to clear area for improved visualization. Often used to clean tissue off bone, e.g., prevertebral tissue in ACDFs, lamina for screw placement, etc.

Varieties: Single or multi-packs.

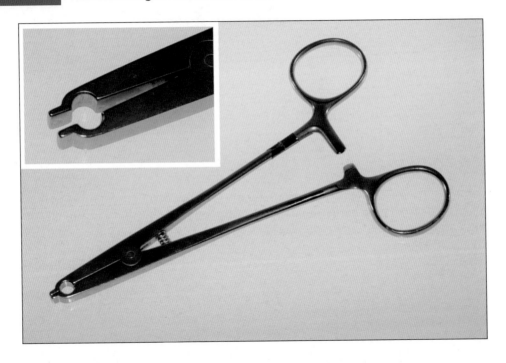

Raney Applier

Alternative Names: Raney clip appliers, skin/scalp clip appliers

Category: General

Purposes: Application of Raney clips to skin flap edges during craniotomy for hemostasis.

Varieties: Reusable or disposable.

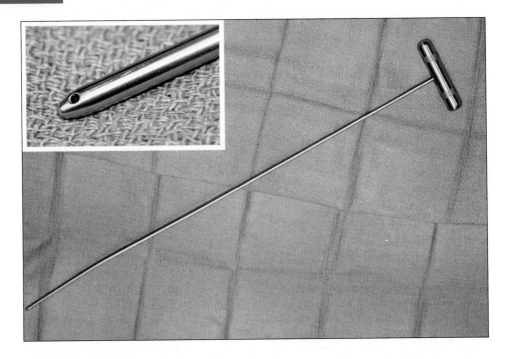

Shunt Passer

Alternative Name: None

Category: General

Purposes: Designed for subcutaneous passage of shunt catheters. Caution is always advised when using this passer, as it can pass through fascia, putting vascular and vital tissue structures at risk of injury. Hole in tip allows catheter to be sutured and secured to passer. Is often accompanied by a plastic sheath. Shorter lengths can also be used to pass electrodes in functional cases or for the creation of subcutaneous tunnels for bypass grafts.

Varieties: Various lengths. Reusable or disposable.

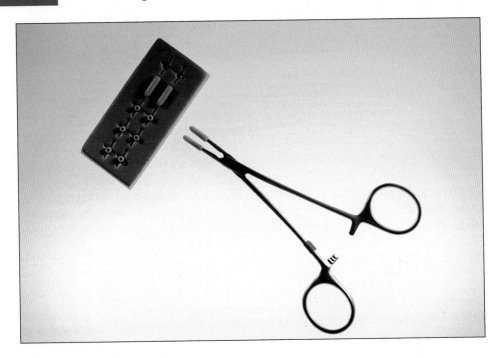

Suture Boots

Alternative Names: Rubber shod, clamp boots, catheter holders

Category: General

Purposes: Small rubber tips for clamps that prevent the serrations from damaging what is being held. Often used to handle shunt or pump catheters. Also used to clamp sutures, since the suture can slip through the serrations of most clamps.

Varieties: Single or multi-packs. Various colors.

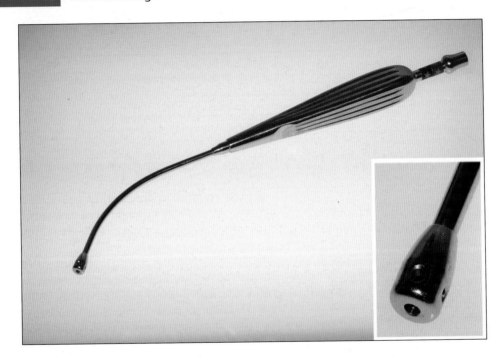

Yankauer Suction

Alternative Name: Tonsil suction tip

Category: General

Purposes: Large-bore suction useful in large surgical exposures. Tip designed to minimize surrounding tissue damage when suctioning.

Varieties: Straight or angled. Protected or non-protected tip. Metal or plastic. Reusable or disposable.

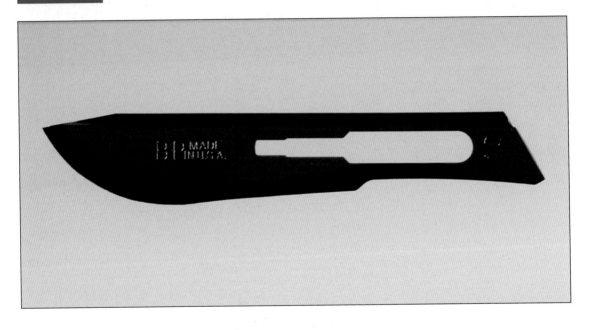

10 Blade

Alternative Name: Skin knife

Category: Blades

Purposes: Large knife blade often used to make skin incisions.

Varieties: None. Various handle types.

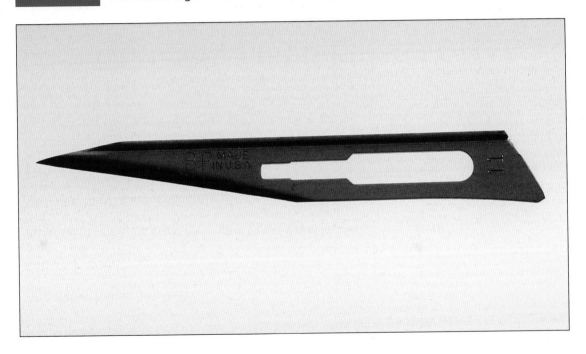

11 Blade

Alternative Name: None

Category: Blades

Purposes: Cutting knife used for fine, precise cutting and dissection of tissues. Often used for initial arteriotomies, opening dura through burr holes, harvesting pericranium, etc. Can be used with the monopolar to make precise holes in the dura when in contact with the monopolar.

Varieties: None. Various handle types.

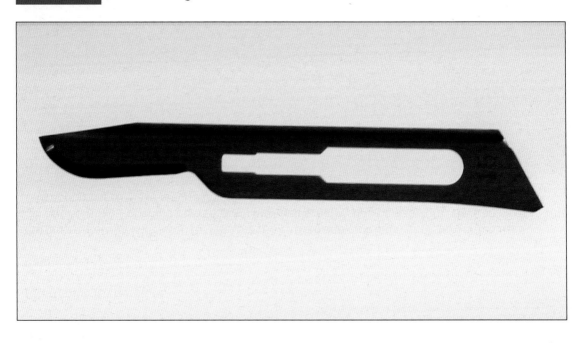

15 Blade

Alternative Name: None

Category: Blades

Purposes: Cutting knife used for fine and precise cutting and dissection of tissues. Often used in pediatrics, skin revisions, harvesting pericranium, and initiating dural incisions.

Varieties: None. Various handle types.

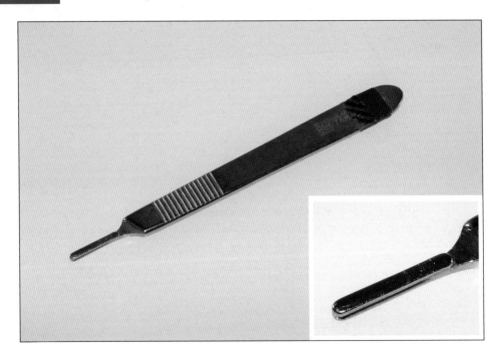

Knife Holder #3

Alternative Name: Often called by the blade type attached

Category: Knife Holders

Purposes: Smaller knife handle used when cutting is required in a small or confined space. Holds 10, 11, 12, and 15 blades.

Varieties: Various shaft lengths.

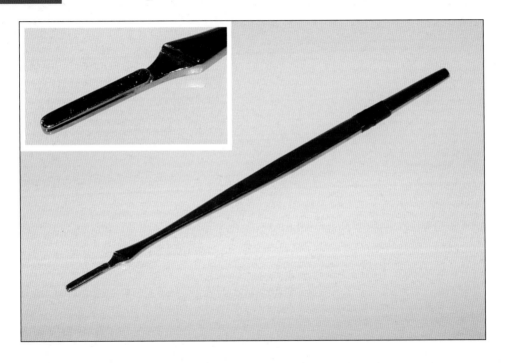

Knife Holder #7

Alternative Name: Often called by the blade type attached

Category: Knife Holders

Purposes: Knife handle used for general cutting needs, most often used for skin incisions. Holds 10, 11, 12, and 15 blades.

Varieties: Various shaft lengths. With and without ruler.

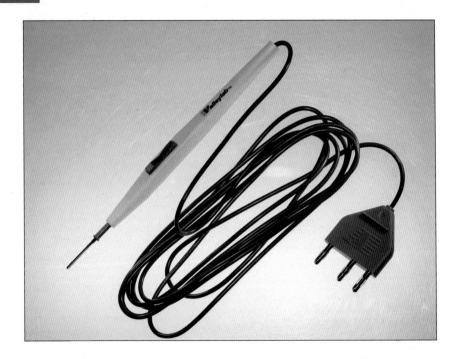

Monopolar

Alternative Names: Bovie, electric knife, cutter, pen knife, cauterizer

Category: Cautery

Purposes: Allows cauterization using high-frequency electrical current through a single electrode that serves as the knife end. The patient's body serves as a ground. Two settings are usually present, one for cutting and the other for cauterization.

Varieties: Universal design. Multiple types of tips, e.g., ring, pinpoint, insulated, etc.

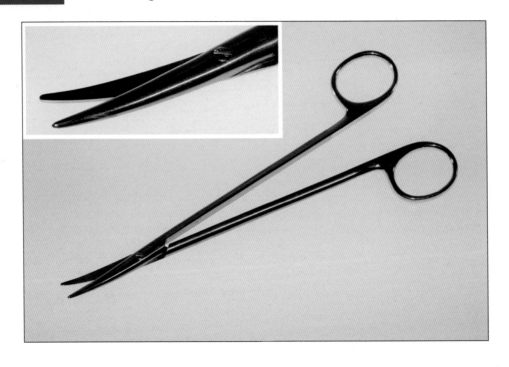

Curved Metzenbaum Scissors

Alternative Names: Metz, curved Metz, Ragnell, tissue scissors, curved tissue scissors

Category: Scissors

Purposes: Useful for macroscopic cutting, dissecting, or undermining delicate soft tissues. Should only be used to cut tissues. Common uses include cutting dura, fascia, ligated vessels, and muscle.

Varieties: Straight or curved blades. Variable lengths of arms.

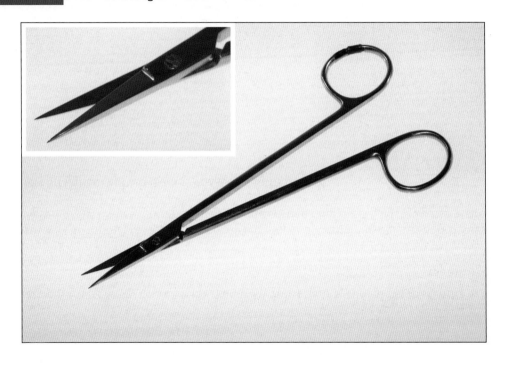

Fine Metzenbaum Scissors

Alternative Names: Metz, fine Metz, fine tissue scissors

Category: Scissors

Purposes: Useful for macroscopic cutting, dissecting, or undermining delicate soft tissues. Should only be used to cut tissues. Common uses include cutting dura, fascia, ligated vessels, and muscle.

Varieties: Straight or curved blades. Variable lengths of arms.

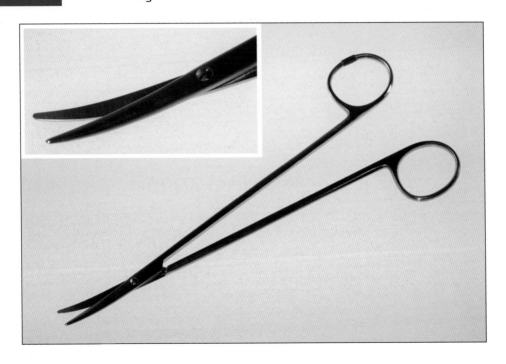

Long Curved Metzenbaum Scissors

Alternative Names: Long Metz, curved Metz, tissue scissors, curved tissue scissors

Category: Scissors

Purposes: Useful for macroscopic cutting, dissecting, or undermining delicate soft tissues. Should only be used to cut tissues. Common uses include cutting dura, fascia, ligated vessels, and muscle.

Varieties: Straight or curved blades. Variable lengths of arms.

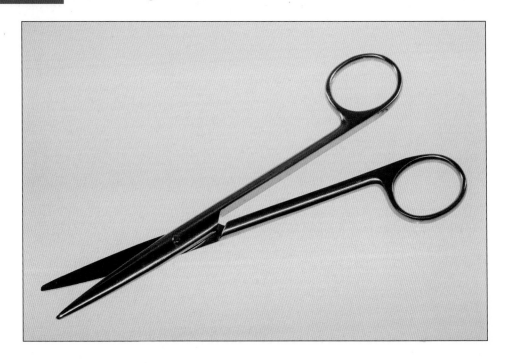

Mayo Scissors

Alternative Name: Suture scissors

Category: Scissors

Purposes: Mainly used for cutting sutures or other non-delicate material.

Varieties: Various lengths of blades and handles.

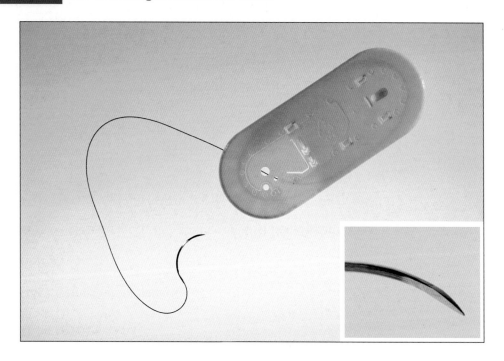

Cutting Suture Needle

Alternative Name: Rarely referred to by their name based on their size

Category: Needles

Purposes: Triangular-shaped needle tip that cuts through tissue as it is placed through tissue.

Varieties: Straight or curved. Various sizes and diameters of the needle. Various types of suture attached.

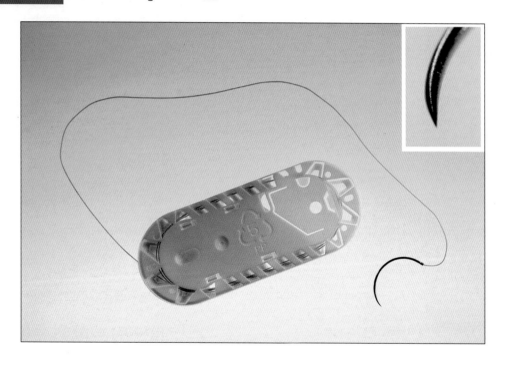

Tapered Suture Needle

Alternative Names: Rarely referred to by their name based on their size

Category: Needles

Purposes: Rounded needle displaces tissue as it is placed through tissue.

Varieties: Straight or curved. Various sizes and diameters of the needle. Various types of suture attached.

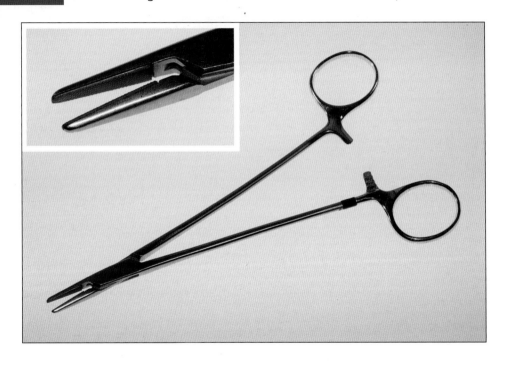

Mayo-Hegar Needle Holder

Alternative Names: Cooley needle holder, DeBakey needle holder, Crile-Wood needle holder, needle driver

Category: Needle holders

Purposes: Locking needle holder used for a multitude of needle sizes. Most common needle holder.

Varieties: Smooth or serrated jaws. Various lengths. Various materials.

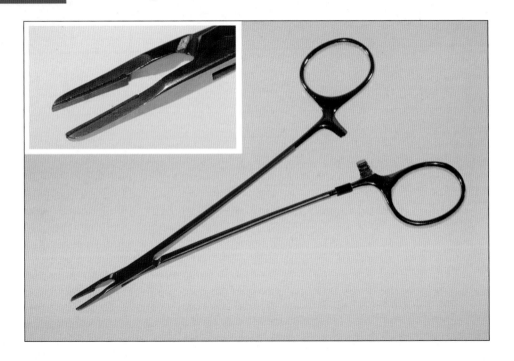

Ryder Needle Holder

Alternative Names: Cooley needle holder, DeBakey needle holder, Crile-Wood needle holder, needle driver

Category: Needle holders

Purposes: Locking needle holder used for a multitude of needle sizes.

Varieties: Smooth or serrated jaws. Various lengths. Various materials.

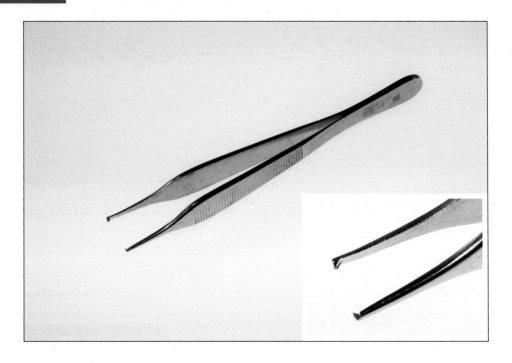

Adson Forceps

Alternative Names: Adson with teeth, Bunny forceps, pickups with teeth, skin forceps, skin pick-ups

Category: Forceps

Purposes: Used for grasping and holding superficial tissues, especially during closing superficial wounds. Allows precise grabbing of skin edges for improved tissue approximation with minimal tissue injury. Sharp teeth can penetrate fragile tissue, surgical materials (shunt valves, catheters), and gloves.

Varieties: The number of teeth, 1×2 or 2×3. No variety in length.

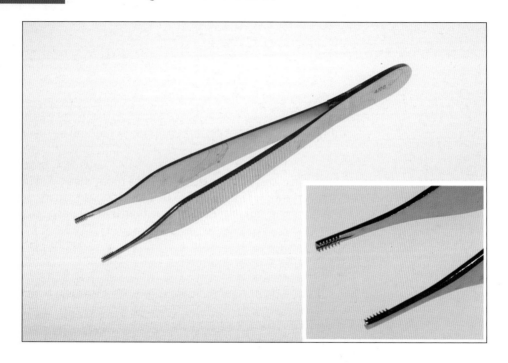

Adson Brown Forceps

Alternative Names: Brown-Adson forceps or pickups, Brown forceps or pickups

Category: Forceps

Purposes: Used for grasping and holding superficial and/or delicate tissues. The interlocking teeth reduce tissue injury. Sharp teeth can penetrate fragile tissue, surgical materials (shunt valves, catheters), and gloves.

Varieties: None.

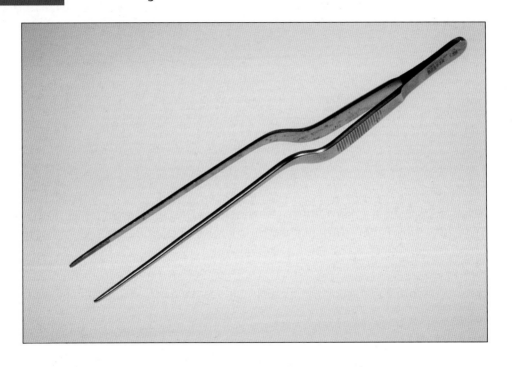

Bayonet Tissue Forceps

Alternative Names: Bayonet, bayonet Cushing, bayonet Cushing tissue forceps, Jansen tissue forceps

Category: Forceps

Purposes: Multitude of uses involving grasping or holding delicate tissue. Allows better visualization of targeted tissue due to bayonet feature. Long arms allow use in deep spaces.

Varieties: Length of arms. The handle will have either a rounded end (Jansen) or edged end (Cushing) that allows scraping abilities.

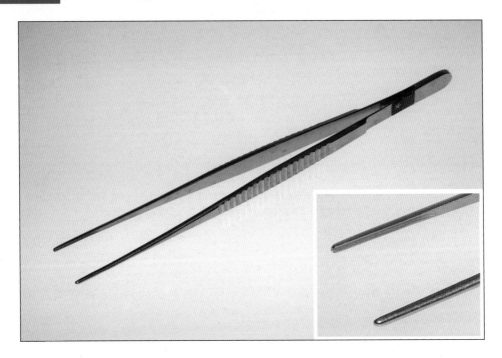

DeBakey Forceps

Alternative Names: DeBakeys, DeBakey pickups, tissue pickups, tissue forceps, vascular forceps, vascular tissue forceps

Category: Forceps

Purposes: Non-traumatic grasping and holding forceps designed for very delicate tissue or vessels. Often used in macroscopic vascular cases. Can also be used for handling tubing and other surgical implants and their cables.

Varieties: Variable instrument lengths.

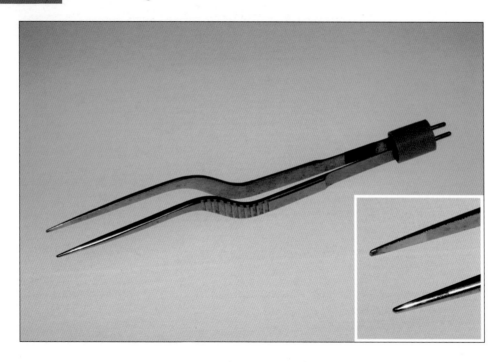

General Bayonet Bipolar Forceps

Alternative Names: Cushing bipolars, Rhoton forceps, Malis bipolars, bayonet, bipolar forceps, bipolars

Category: Forceps

Purposes: Coagulation of tissue between the tips of the forceps, which must be in close contact to allow current to flow through tissue. Variable current allows highly tailored effectiveness. Can be used as a dissection instrument or for general grasping of delicate tissues.

Varieties: Straight, curved, or angled tips. Insulated tips or not. Irrigating or not. Short and long. Blunt or fine tips.

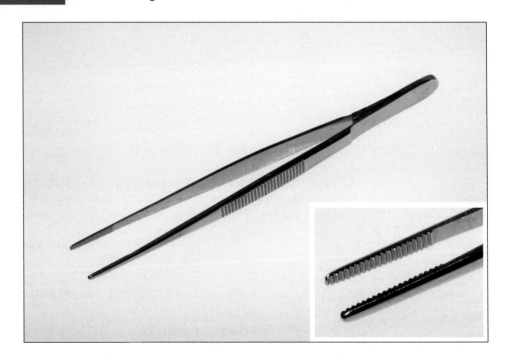

General Tissue Forceps

Alternative Names: Cushing forceps, Semken forceps, forceps without teeth, smooth forceps

Category: Forceps

Purposes: Multipurpose atraumatic forceps used for grasping, holding, retracting, countertraction, and stabilizing various tissue types.

Varieties: Various lengths.

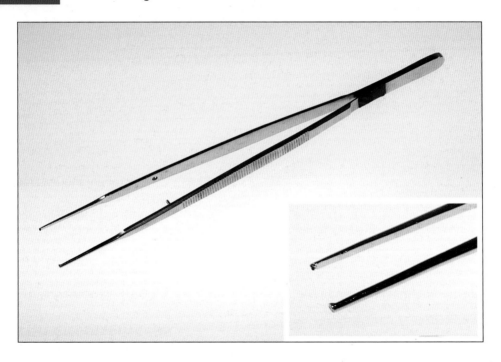

Gerald with Teeth

Alternative Names: Pickups with teeth, Gerald with, Cushing with teeth (incorrect)

Category: Forceps

Purposes: Grasping and holding forceps designed for very delicate tissue or vessels. Great for holding hearty tissue, e.g., dura, fascia, etc., for stabilization during suturing or retraction.

Varieties: None.

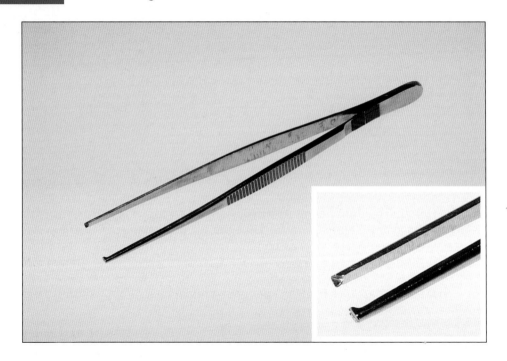

Large Tissue Forceps

Alternative Names: Semken forceps with teeth, rat tooth forceps, forceps with teeth

Category: Forceps

Purposes: Multipurpose sharp-toothed forceps used for grasping, holding, retracting, countertraction, and stabilizing moderate to heavy tissue types. Most often used in wound closures, except not directly on the skin.

Varieties: Various lengths.

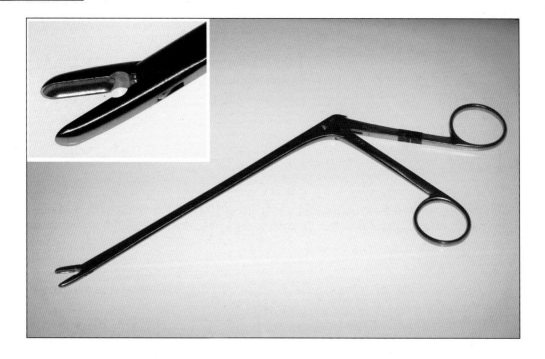

Takahashi Forceps

Alternative Names: Pituitary, tissue forceps

Category: Forceps

Purposes: Grasping and manipulating tissue during endonasal/transsphenoidal cases. Can be used for tissue grasping and biopsy samples in cranial and spinal cases.

Varieties: Straight or angled jaws. Various jaw sizes. Variable length of instrument.

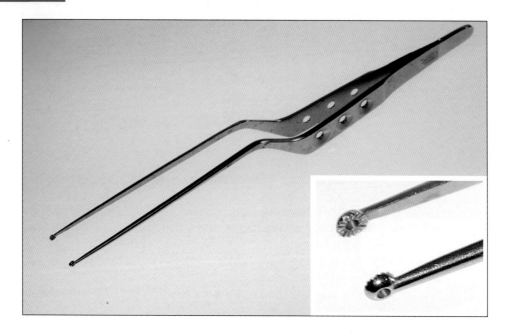

Yasargil Bayonet Tissue Forceps

Alternative Names: Bayonet, bayonet Cushing, bayonet Cushing tissue forceps, Jansen tissue forceps

Category: Forceps

Purposes: Multitude of uses involving grasping or holding delicate tissue. Cupped jaws allow more secure tissue purchase. Long arms allow use in deep spaces. Good for grasping biopsy samples and fat grafts.

Varieties: Length of arms. Size of jaws.

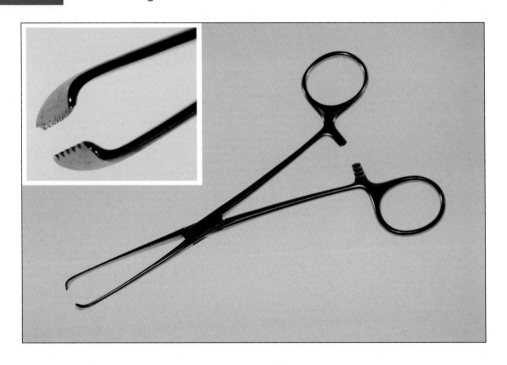

Allis Clamp

Alternative Names: Clamp with teeth, tissue clamp

Category: Clamps

Purposes: Used in securing, lifting or holding masses or tissue destined for resection, e.g., spinal lipoma, large intracranial meningioma, or fat for fat graft. The interlocking teeth reduce tissue injury. Also used for securing cords, cables, and suction tubing to the surgical drapes.

Varieties: The number of teeth, 4×5, 5×6, or 9×10. May be curved or straight and come in a variety of lengths.

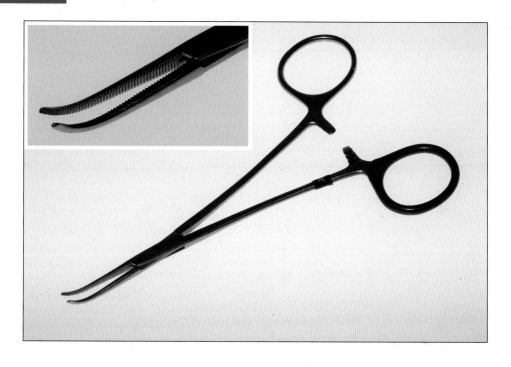

Classic Clamp

Alternative Names: Clamp, Crile clamp, Lahey clamp, Halstead clamp, Adson clamp, Mixter clamp, obtuse clamp, snap, hemostat

Category: Clamps

Purposes: Clamping or occluding vessels or delicate tissue. Used also to dissect tissue planes. Used commonly to grasp and occlude vessels. May be used to pass a suture tie around occluded vessels. Also can be used to secure items to the surgical drape.

Varieties: Straight, curved, and angled. Variable lengths of handles.

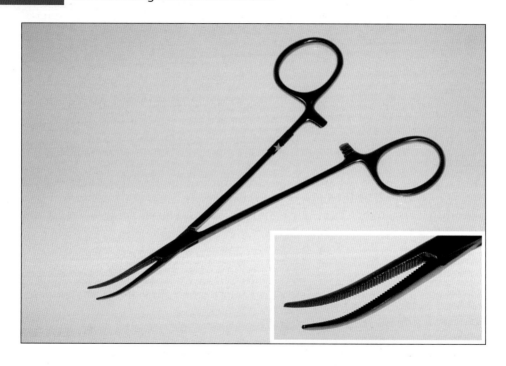

Crile Clamp

Alternative Names: Clamp, Lahey clamp, Halstead clamp, Adson clamp, Mixter clamp, obtuse clamp, snap, hemostat

Category: Clamps

Purposes: The most commonly used clamp. Clamping or occluding vessels or delicate tissue. Used also to dissect tissue planes. Used commonly to grasp and occlude vessels. Also can be used to secure items to the surgical drape.

Varieties: Straight, curved, and angled. Variable lengths of handles.

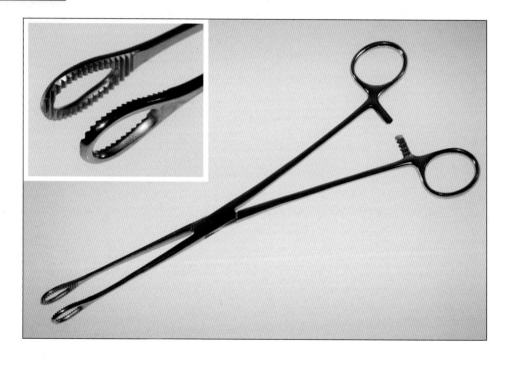

Foerster Sponge Stick

Alternative Names: Sponge stick, ringed forceps, Fletcher sponge stick (incorrect)

Category: Clamps

Purposes: Large forceps good for grasping and holding tissues. Most commonly used with a 4×4 mounted, and used for surgical prepping, blunt dissection, and improving visualization by soaking up blood in large wounds.

Varieties: Straight or curved. Variable lengths of arms. Smooth or serrated jaws.

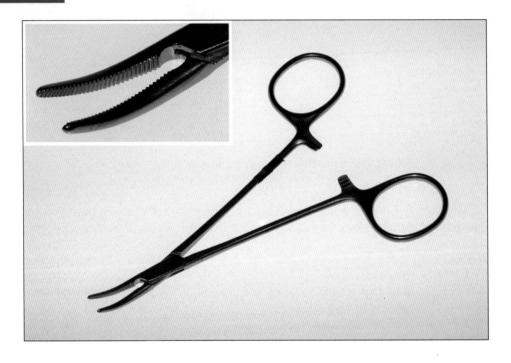

Halstead Mosquito Clamp

Alternative Names: Clamp, mosquito, Halstead, Hartman, hemostat, mini snap, snap

Category: Clamps

Purposes: Often used for clamping or occluding vessels and/or delicate tissue. Also can be used to secure items to the surgical drape or to hold sutured tissues for retraction, e.g., dura.

Varieties: Straight or curved jaws.

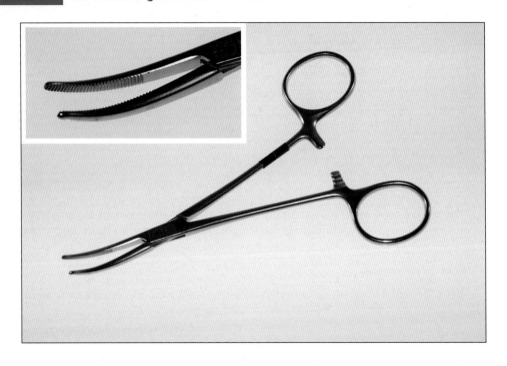

Kelly Clamp

Alternative Names: Clamp, Crile clamp, Rochester clamp, Pean clamp, hemostat

Category: Clamps

Purposes: The most commonly used clamp. Used to clamp or occlude vessels or delicate tissue. Used also to dissect tissue planes. Used commonly to grasp and occlude vessels. Also can be used to secure items to the surgical drape.

Varieties: Straight, curved, and angled. Variable lengths of handles.

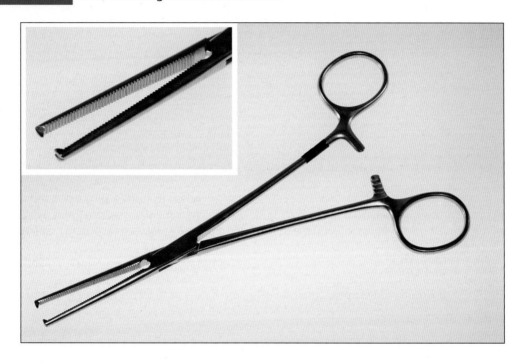

Kocher Clamp

Alternative Names: Koch clamp, Ochsner clamp, Rochester-Ochsner clamp, clamp with teeth, bone clamp

Category: Clamps

Purposes: Used in securing, lifting, or holding masses or tissue destined for resection, e.g., spinal lipoma, large intracranial meningioma, fat for fat graft, and fascia for approximation. Also used for stabilizing bony fragments, e.g., fibula for graft molding, spinous processes for lifting and removal, etc.

Varieties: Straight or curved jaws. Variable lengths.

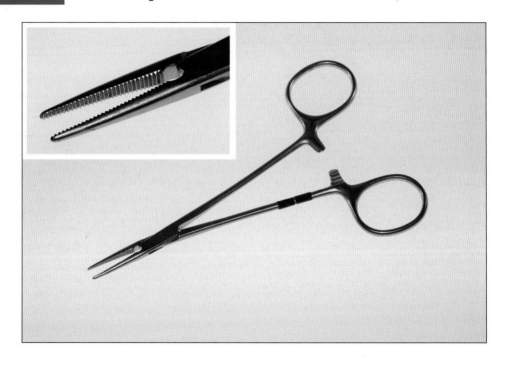

Straight Halstead Mosquito Clamp

Alternative Names: Clamp, mosquito, Halstead, Hartman, hemostat, mini snap, snap

Category: Clamps

Purposes: Often used for clamping or occluding vessels and/or delicate tissue. Also can be used to secure items to the surgical drape or to hold sutured tissues for retraction, e.g., dura.

Varieties: Straight or curved jaws.

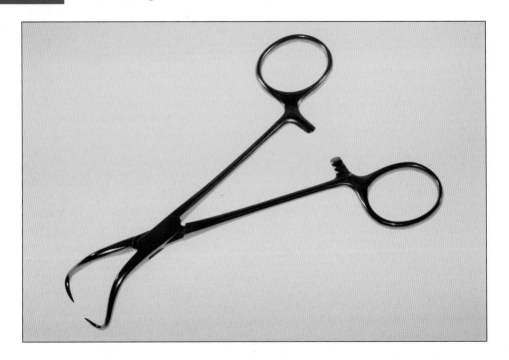

Towel Clamps

Alternative Names: Backhaus clamp, Edna clamp, Jones clamp, Peers towel clamp

Category: Clamps

Purposes: Multipurpose instrument for securing items to surgical drapes, grasping thick tissue, tumor, or bone for retraction or countertraction.

Varieties: Perforating/non-perforating or sharp/blunt ends. Variable lengths of arms. Hinged or spring self-retaining mechanism.

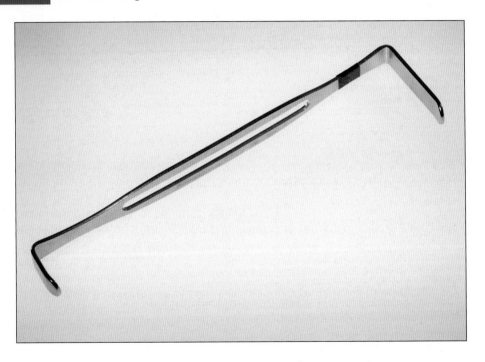

Army-Navy Retractor

Alternative Names: US, Army, US Army, or Navy retractor

Category: Retractors

Purposes: Maintaining retraction in small wounds. Alternatively, these retractors can be used to push tissue out of the way as well. Good for anterior fat harvest, initial parts of MIS (posterior and lateral) cases, and functional implant cases.

Varieties: None.

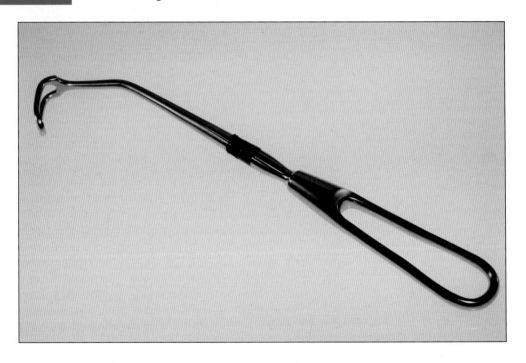

Cushing Retractor

Alternative Names: Curved tissue retractor, Cushing nerve retractor, curved Cushing retractor

Category: Retractors

Purposes: Retraction of skin or muscle flaps, especially during craniotomies. Also used when making burr holes for protection from surrounding tissue interference by pushing away tissue and placing the drill bit within the curve of the instrument tip.

Varieties: None.

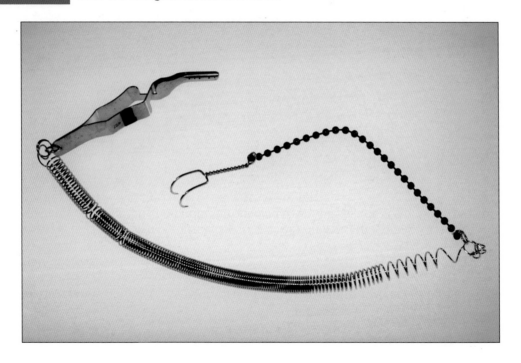

Fish hooks with Songer cables

Alternative Names: Fish hooks, flap hooks, dural fish hooks, Songer hooks

Category: Retractors

Purposes: Retraction of skin, muscle, or dural flaps. The hooks attach to cables (springed or not), which are secured to the drapes. Minimally traumatic retraction system for craniotomy flaps.

Varieties: Sharp or dull hooks. Springed or not cables. Single or double hooks.

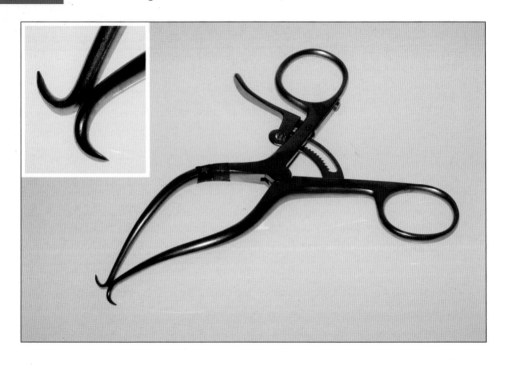

Gelpi Retractor

Alternative Names: Angled Gelpi, short Gelpi

Category: Retractors

Purposes: Used for retraction of surface tissue to allow for improved visualization of the surrounding area. Sharp ends provide point retraction of wound. Used throughout neurosurgical procedures for superficial and deep tissue retraction.

Varieties: Curved and angled ends. Various lengths. Locking and not.

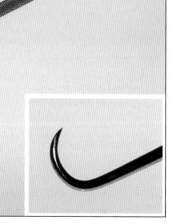

Joseph Skin Hooks

Alternative Names: Cottle skin hook, Gilles skin hook, Freer skin hook, skin hook, single hook

Category: Retractors

Purposes: Retraction of skin and muscle for increasing wound exposure. Useful for holding pericranium during harvesting or for holding up skin flaps.

Varieties: Sharp or blunt hook. Various lengths.

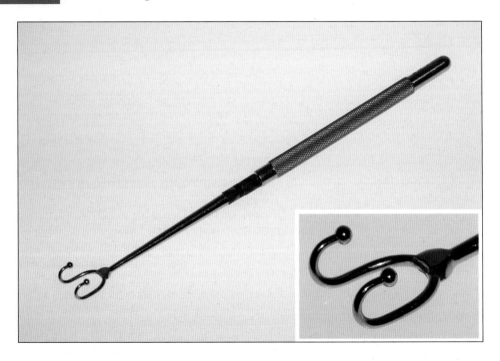

Joseph Skin Hooks 2-Prong

Alternative Names: Blunt Joseph hook, blunt Cottle double hook, skin hook

Category: Retractors

Purposes: Retraction of skin and muscle for increasing wound exposure. Useful for holding pericranium during harvesting or for holding up skin flaps.

Varieties: Various lengths.

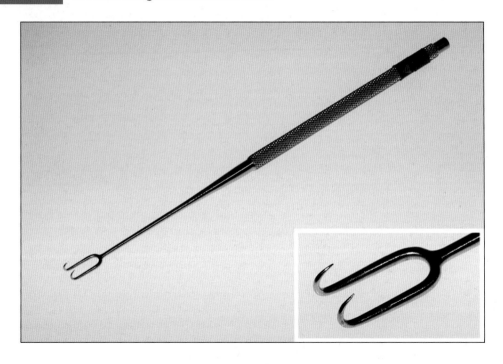

Joseph Skin Hooks 2-Prong Sharp

Alternative Names: Joseph hook, Guthrie hook, Cottle double hook, skin hook

Category: Retractors

Purposes: Retraction of skin and muscle for increasing wound exposure. Useful for holding pericranium during harvesting or for holding up skin flaps.

Varieties: Various lengths.

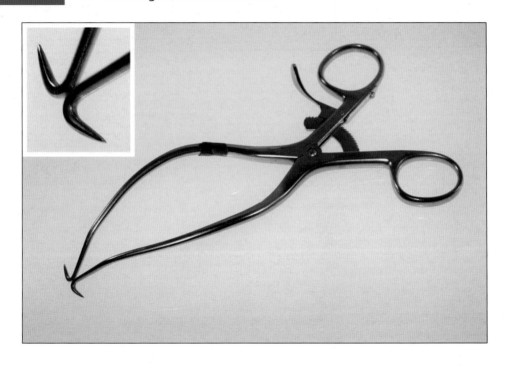

Long Gelpi Retractor

Alternative Names: Angled Gelpi, short Gelpi

Category: Retractors

Purposes: Used for retraction of surface tissue to allow for improved visualization of the surrounding area. Sharp ends provide point retraction of wound. Used throughout neurosurgical procedures for superficial and deep tissue retraction.

Varieties: Curved and angled ends. Various lengths. Locking and not.

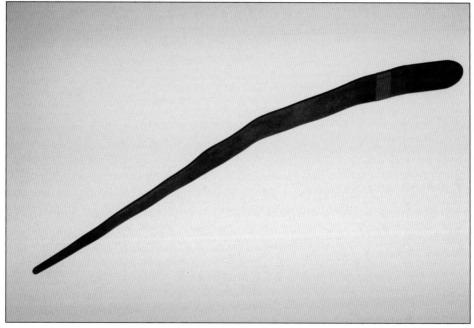

Malleable Brain Retractor

Alternative Names: Malleable retractor, brain ribbon, brain retractor

Category: Retractors

Purposes: Flexible handheld or mountable brain retractor. Can be shaped for custom retraction angles.

Varieties: Various widths, shapes, and materials.

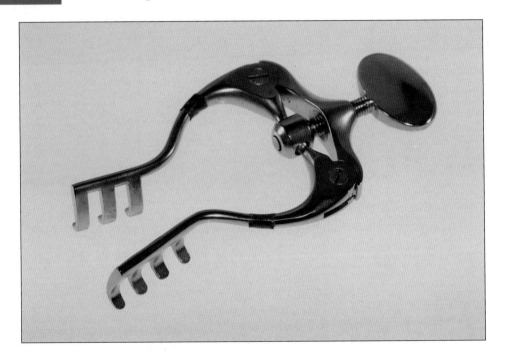

Mastoid Retractor

Alternative Names: Jansen-mastoid, Weitlaner-Mollison, Weitlaner, small Weitlaner, mastoid

Category: Retractors

Purposes: Self-retaining retraction system for skin and soft tissue. Can be used for any small skin incisions, percutaneous screw placement, or any other procedure utilizing only small incisions.

Varieties: Straight, curved, or angled arms. Sharp or blunt teeth. Single or multi-toothed jaws.

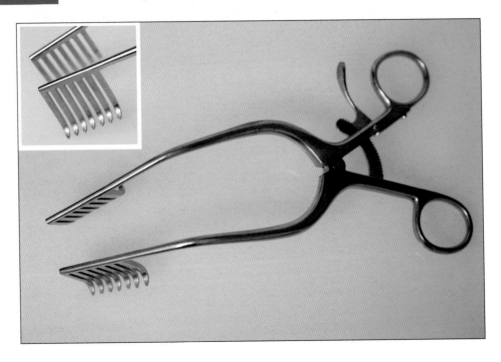

Miskimon Retractor

Alternative Names: D'Errico-Adson, Mollison, curved Weitlaner, curved cerebellar

Category: Retractors

Purposes: Self-retaining retraction of skin and soft tissue, especially in larger and deeper wounds, particularly spine and posterior fossa cases.

Varieties: Sharp or blunt teeth. Single or multi-toothed jaws.

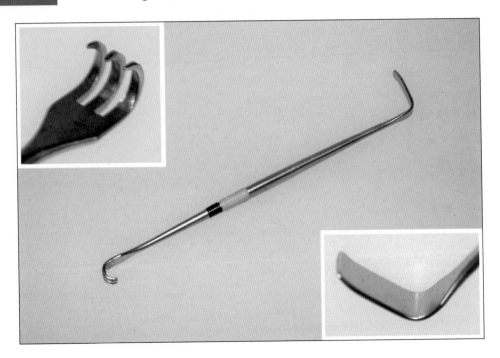

Senn Retractor

Alternative Names: Miller-Senn, skin rake, rake

Category: Retractors

Purposes: Double-ended instrument for retraction of skin and muscle for increasing wound exposure. Useful for holding pericranium during harvesting or for holding up skin flaps. Also good for retracting small amounts of tissue or skin in confined spaces.

Varieties: Sharp or blunt teeth.

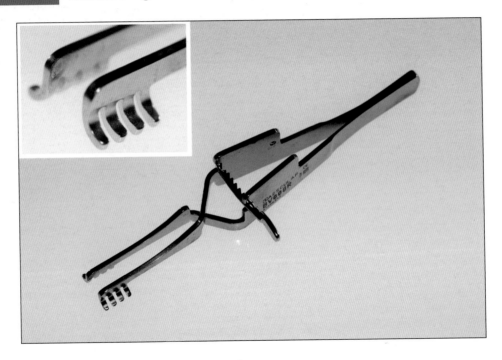

Small Toothed Retractor

Alternative Names: Heiss retractor, wound spreader, small skin retractor

Category: Retractors

Purposes: Used for retraction of small openings in the skin. Can be used for any burr holes, percutaneous screw placement, or any other procedure utilizing only small incisions.

Varieties: Single or multi-toothed jaws.

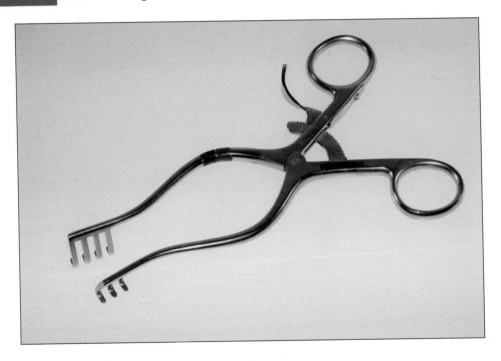

Weitlaner Retractor

Alternative Names: D'Errico-Adson, Mollison, cerebellar, curved cerebellar

Category: Retractors

Purposes: Self-retaining retraction of skin and soft tissue. One of the most common retractors used in neurosurgery.

Varieties: Sharp or blunt teeth. Single or multi-toothed jaws.

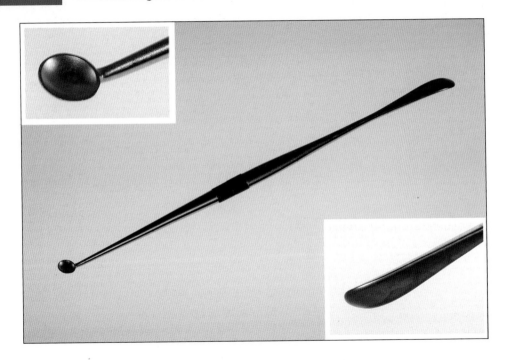

Penfield #1

Alternative Names: Number 1, large pancake dissector

Category: Dissectors

Purposes: Double-ended instrument for dissecting, scraping, and separating soft tissue from bone, e.g., nasal septum, skull base, dura, etc., and even as a protection device when drilling. The blunt end is smaller and less curved than the Penfield 2 but still can be used to separate bone from dura.

Varieties: None.

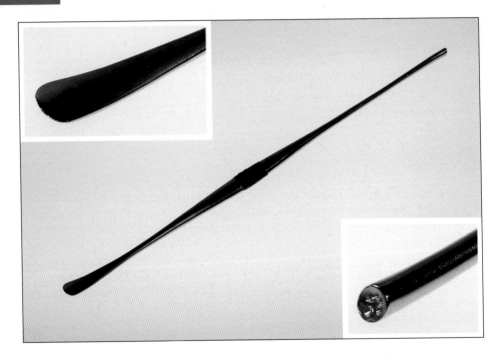

Penfield #2

Alternative Name: Two dissector

Category: Dissectors

Purposes: Double-ended instrument for dissecting, scraping, and separating soft tissue from bone, e.g., nasal septum, skull base, dura, etc., and even as a protection device when drilling or placing bone wax for hemostasis in narrow spaces. The blunt end is less curved than the Penfield 3 but still can be used to separate bone from dura.

Varieties: None.

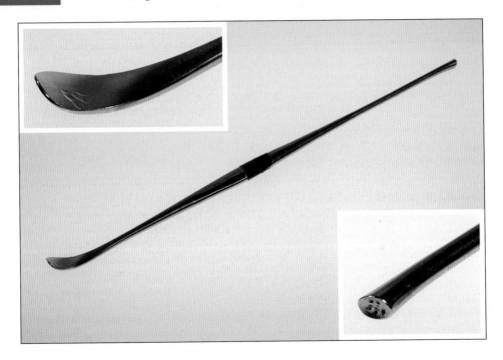

Penfield #3

Alternative Name: Three dissector

Category: Dissectors

Purposes: Double-ended instrument for dissecting, scraping, and separating soft tissue from bone, e.g., nasal septum, skull base, dura, etc., and even as a protection device when drilling or placing bone wax for hemostasis in narrow spaces. The curved end is most often used to separate bone from dura through burr holes.

Varieties: None.

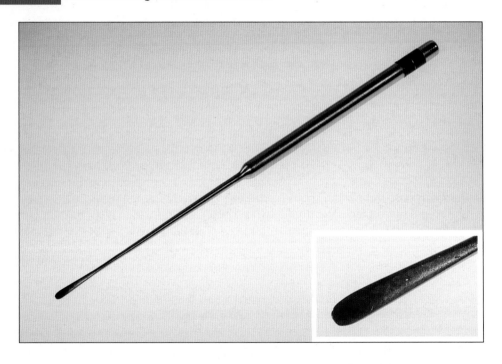

Penfield #4

Alternative Name: Four dissector

Category: Dissectors

Purposes: Multipurpose tool used for dissecting and scraping. Frequent uses include separating soft tissue from bone, e.g., nasal septum, skull base, dura, etc., and even as a protection device when drilling or placing bone wax for hemostasis in narrow spaces. Also used for deepening corticectomy incisions and exploration for intraparenchymal hematomas. The back of the handle can also be used to place bone wax in particular areas, e.g., screw holes, bleeding bone edges, etc., for hemostasis.

Varieties: None.

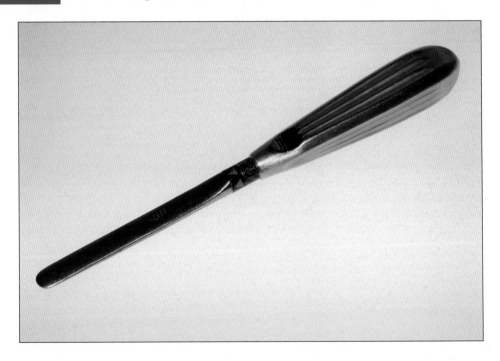

Boles Elevator

Alternative Names: Periosteal, Langenbeck elevator (incorrect), Cobb elevator (incorrect)

Category: Elevators

Purposes: Scraping tissue off fascia and bone, e.g., periosteum. Can also be used to retract or protect soft tissue when drilling through bone (dural tack-up sutures during craniotomy).

Varieties: Sharp/blunt or narrow/wide ends. Curved or straight. Variable length of shaft.

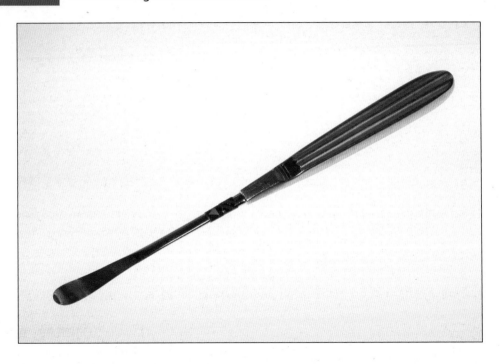

Cottle Crani Elevator

Alternative Names: Periosteal, Cobb elevator

Category: Elevators

Purposes: Scraping tissue, in particular periosteum and dura, off bone. Can also be used to retract or protect soft tissue when drilling through bone (dural tack-up sutures during craniotomy).

Varieties: Sharp/blunt or narrow/wide ends. Curved or straight. Variable length of shaft.

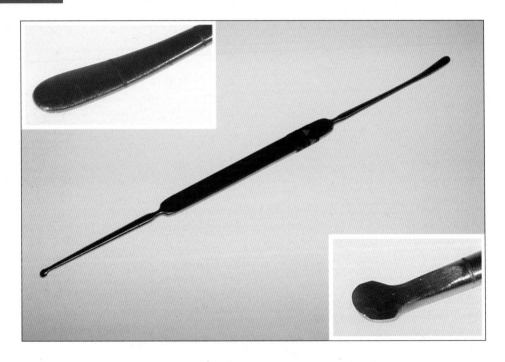

Cottle Elevator

Alternative Names: Septal elevator, mucosa elevator

Category: Elevators

Purposes: Double-ended instrument with a sharp, flat end and the other with a teardrop shape, allowing the dissection of delicate soft tissue off, most commonly, the septum. However, it can be used to separate the dura, ligament, or other soft tissue from bone.

Varieties: None.

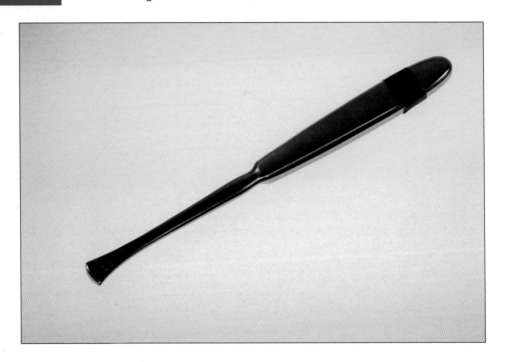

Langenbeck Elevator

Alternative Names: Periosteal, Cottle crani elevator, Chandler elevator, Cobb elevator

Category: Elevators

Purposes: Very useful in scraping tissue off both fascia and bone, in particular periosteum. Can also be used to retract or protect soft tissue when drilling through bone (dural tack-up sutures during craniotomy).

Varieties: Sharp/blunt or narrow/wide ends. Curved or straight. Variable length of shaft.

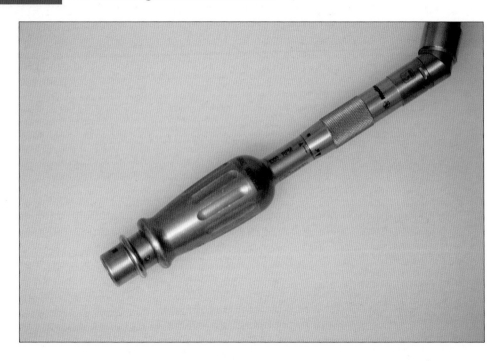

Drill Handle

Alternative Name: Dependent on the drill bit attached

Category: Drills

Purposes: Mechanism for housing drill bits and attachments.

Varieties: Pneumatic or electric power source. Ergonomic or more cylindrical housing. Straight or curved.

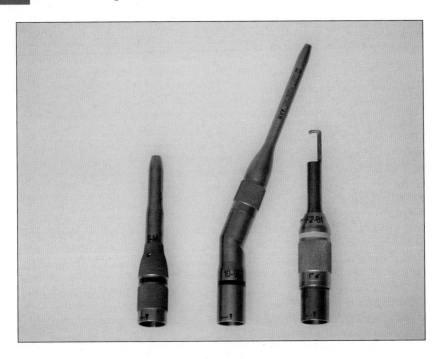

Drill Handle Attachments

Alternative Name: Dependent on the drill bit attached

Category: Drills

Purposes: Drill attachment that is held by the operator. Various attachments to accommodate variable drill bits. Guarded tips usually reserved for craniotome while open-ended tips can accommodate other bits, such as diamond burr, acorn, or screw tip bits.

Varieties: Straight or curved. Open-ended or guarded.

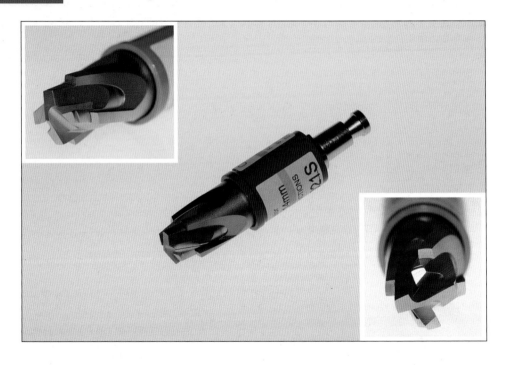

Perforator Drill Bit

Alternative Name: Burr hole bit

Category: Bits

Purposes: Used for placement of burr holes. Spring-loaded bit releases upon experiencing low resistance, resulting in cessation of drilling.

Varieties: Various diameters of cutting bit.

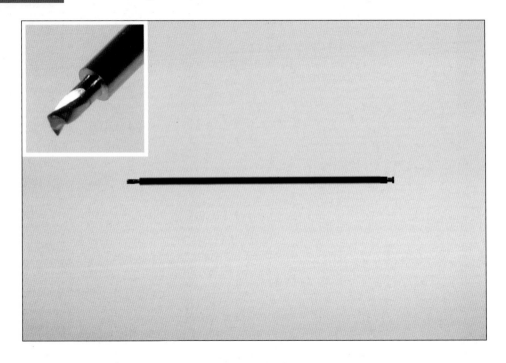

Twist Drill Bit

Alternative Names: Twist drill, screw bit, tap

Category: Bits

Purposes: Tapping holes in bone before screw placement.

Varieties: Various diameters and lengths of bit.

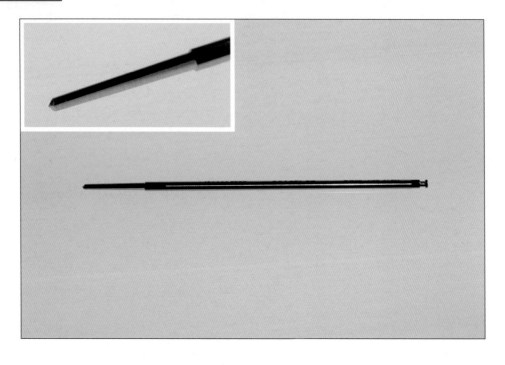

Craniotome Bit

Alternative Names: Footed bit, tapered bit, tapered spiral bit

Category: Bits

Purposes: Usually used with protective footplate that protects the drill bit from tissue below. Most often used to cut bone between burr holes, to make limited and specific lamina cuts, and to perform other types of custom bone work. Without the footplate, this bit can be used to make holes in bone, e.g., the bone flap for sutures, so long as the bit is protected from soft tissue by other means.

Varieties: Various diameters and lengths of bit.

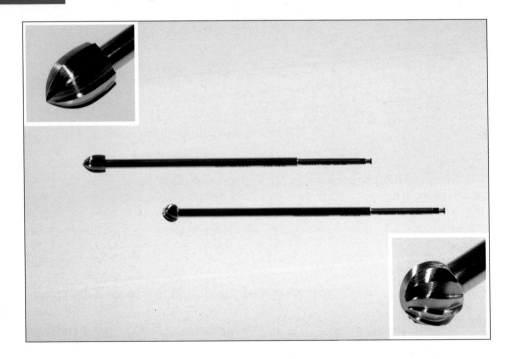

Cutting Drill Bits

Alternative Names: Fluted ball, acorn, round cutter

Category: Bits

Purposes: Allows removal of large amounts of bone in a short amount of time through coarse drilling. Can also be used to thin out bone in preparation for punch removal. Caution should be used around delicate structures, as these drill bits have no protective features when they come into contact with tissue.

Varieties: Various sizes and shapes of drill bit.

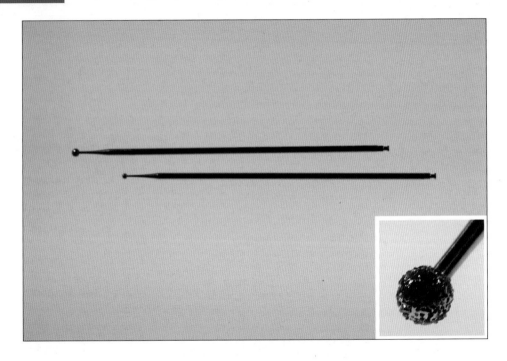

Diamond Burr

Alternative Names: Diamond, coarse diamond bit

Category: Bits

Purposes: Drill bit that allows more precise drilling but requires more time and generates more heat. Often used when drilling around vital structures and in more confined spaces, e.g., clinoidectomies, transverse foramina, etc. Heat generated can be used for hemostasis in more vascularized bone, e.g., sphenoid ridge. Otherwise, copious irrigation is recommended.

Varieties: Fine or coarse bits. Various diameters. Various lengths of the shaft. Various materials.

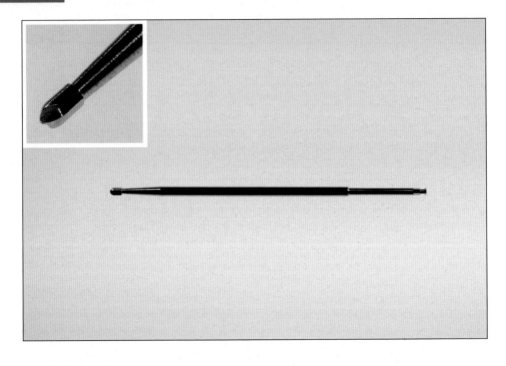

Match Head Drill Bit

Alternative Name: Tapered side cutting, M8

Category: Bits

Purposes: Drill bit that allows precision drilling in a side-to-side fashion. The bit is designed not to cut when placed directly on top of structures. Often used for trimming or removing small amounts of undesired bone or thinning out bone above vital structures.

Varieties: Various diameters and lengths of bit.

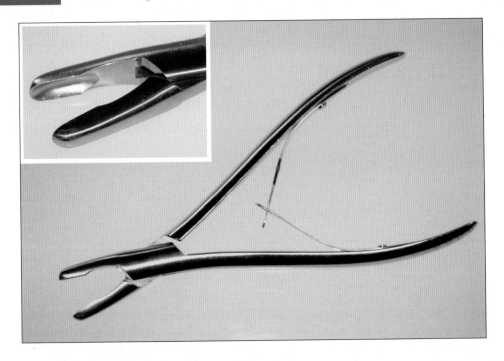

Adson Rongeur

Alternative Names: Bone rongeur, Juers-Lempert or Lempert rongeur (although incorrect), aneurysm rongeur or bone cutter

Category: Rongeurs

Purposes: Removal of bone and soft tissue, often used for removing temporal squamous bone, sphenoid wing, and occipital bone.

Varieties: None.

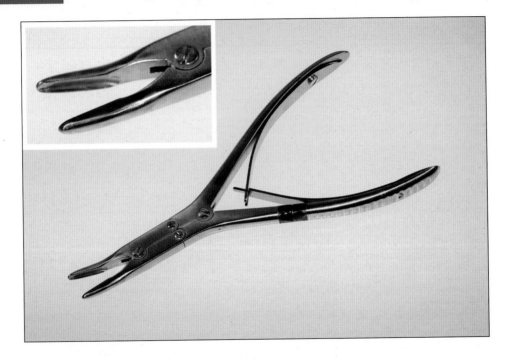

Beyer Rongeur

Alternative Names: Bone rongeur, Ruskin rongeur, small double-action rongeur

Category: Rongeurs

Purposes: Removal of bone and soft tissue. Often used for removing temporal squamous bone, sphenoid wing, and occipital bone. Also good for removing calcified tissue or other adherent soft tissue in open spine cases.

Varieties: Straight or curved jaws. Variable sized cups at the tips.

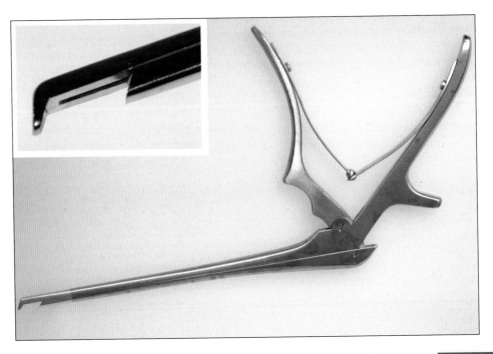

Kerrison Rongeur

Alternative Names: Ruggles, punch, spine rongeur, up or down biting rongeur

Category: Rongeurs

Purposes: Allows precise bone removal by guillotine cutting of small pieces of bone and soft tissue, e.g., ligaments. Foot plate allows stabilization or non-traumatic placement of instrument over vital tissue.

Varieties: Up or down biting. 40°, 45°, or 90° angled tip. Various widths of biting jaw. Coated or non-coated.

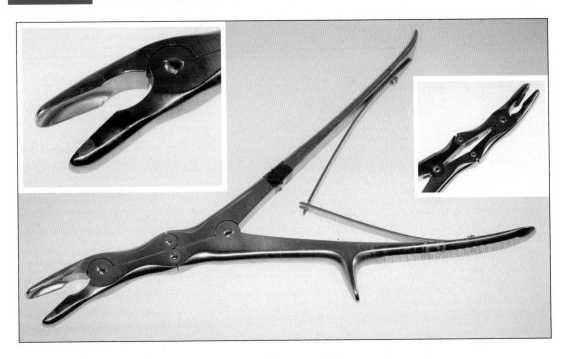

Leksell Stille Rongeur

Alternative Names: Leksell, double-action, large rongeur, Beyer rongeur (incorrect), Luer-Echlin rongeur (incorrect), Sklar-Ruskin rongeur (incorrect), Adson rongeur (incorrect)

Category: Rongeurs

Purposes: Double-action bone rongeur used for removal of bone and soft tissue. Often used for removing temporal squamous bone, sphenoid wing, spinous processes, lamina, and osteophytes, and for shaping bone flaps. Double action allows more force to be applied to bone.

Varieties: Straight or curved jaws. Variable width of jaws.

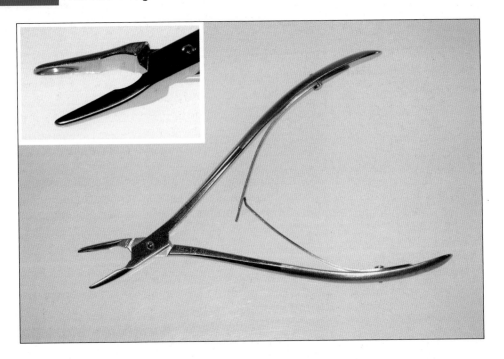

Lempert Rongeur

Alternative Names: Small bone rongeur, Adson rongeur (incorrect), Luer-Friedman, Juers-Lempert, aneurysm rongeur, small bone cutter

Category: Rongeurs

Purposes: Single-action rongeur good for removing small amounts of soft tissue and bone. Often used in confined spaces, e.g., along sphenoid ridge during pterional craniotomies, small amounts of C1 lamina in posterior fossa cases, etc.

Varieties: None.

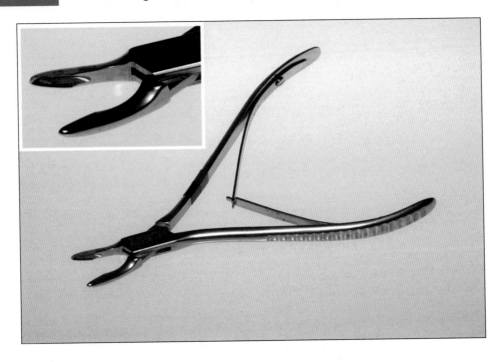

Luer Friedmann Rongeur

Alternative Names: Small bone rongeur, Adson rongeur (incorrect), Juers-Lempert, Lempert rongeur, aneurysm rongeur, small bone cutter

Category: Rongeurs

Purposes: Single-action rongeur good for removing small amounts of soft tissue and bone. Often used in confined spaces, e.g., along sphenoid ridge during pterional craniotomies, small amounts of C1 lamina in posterior fossa cases, etc.

Varieties: None.

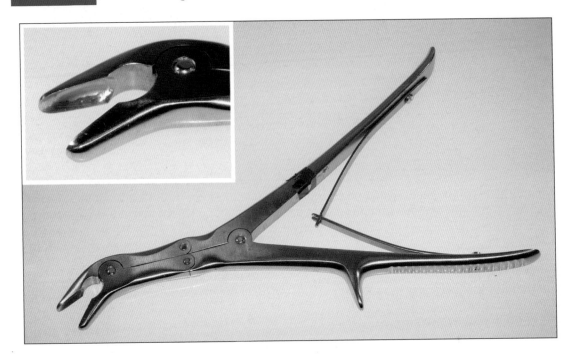

Stille Rongeur

Alternative Names: Duckbill, Sklar-Stille rongeur, Leksell (incorrect), double-action, Beyer rongeur (incorrect), Sklar-Ruskin rongeur (incorrect), Adson rongeur (incorrect)

Category: Rongeurs

Purposes: Double-action bone rongeur used for removal of bone and soft tissue. Often used for removing temporal squamous bone, sphenoid wing, spinous processes, lamina, and osteophytes, and for shaping bone flaps. Double action allows more force to be applied to bone. More narrow jaws allow bone biting in more confined spaces.

Varieties: None.

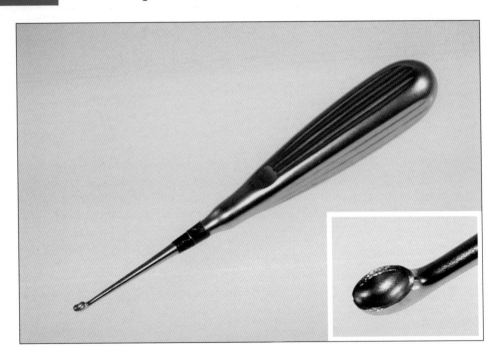

Volkmann Bone Curette

Alternative Names: Spine curette, Brun, bone, oval, round, straight/curved curette

Category: Curettes

Purposes: Multipurpose instrument good for scraping tissue off bone (lateral recess and ligament), debriding and removing debris, and/or harvesting bone. Curved curettes are used to free or separate disc fragments and can also be used as dural separators.

Varieties: Straight or angled varieties. The angles can be right, left, upgoing, downgoing, etc. Multiple sizes for cutting end. Can be open or cupped. Various lengths of shaft.

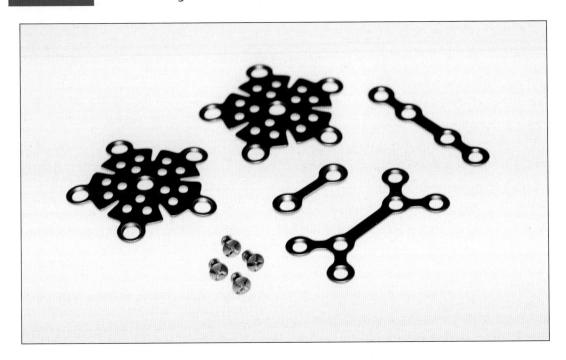

Cranial Plates

Alternative Names: Fixation plates, plates, burr hole covers, dog bone, or other named plate

Category: Cranial Plates

Purposes: Used to join bony surfaces together, most often used to affix a bone plate, plate lamina or zygoma, or other bone surfaces to be joined together.

Varieties: Various shapes and sizes of plates and screws.

Chapter 5: Basic Microsurgical/Microvascular/Skull Base Instrumentation

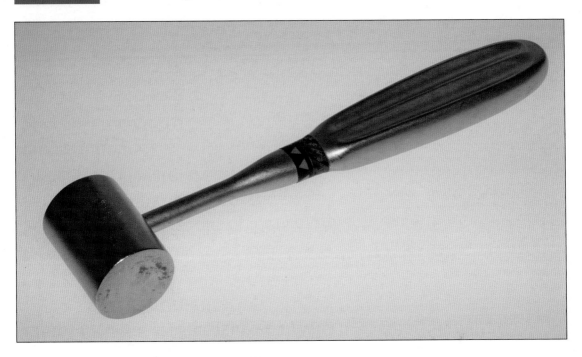

Cottle Mallet

Alternative Names: Mallet, hammer

Category: General

Purposes: Used for application of force, usually on another instrument, e.g., osteotome, bone graft impactor, chisel, etc.

Varieties: Variable weights. Variable material of mallet and handle.

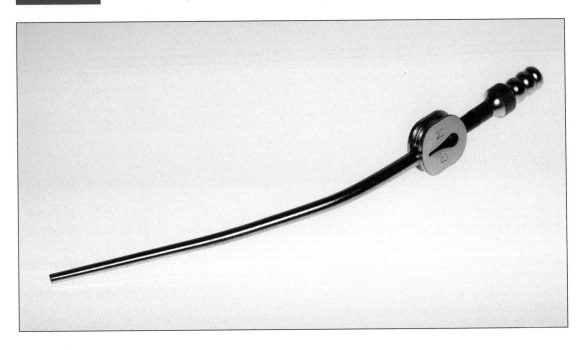

Japanese Suction

Alternative Names: Fukishima, variable suction, regulated suction tip

Category: General

Purposes: Used for suction of fluids in confined spaces. Teardrop-shaped thumb hole allows regulated style of suction. Also used as a retractor, protection device, and blunt dissection tool when removing tumor or brain parenchyma.

Varieties: Straight or angled. Various diameters of tips.

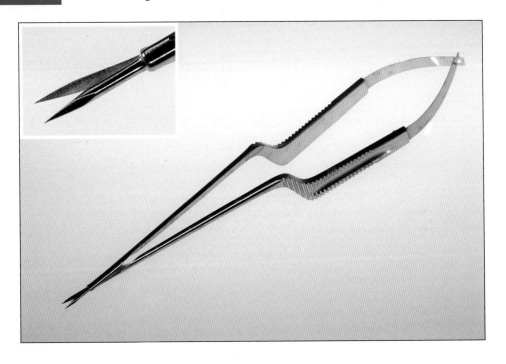

Bayonet Micro Scissors

Alternative Names: Yasargil micro scissors, micro scissors

Category: Scissors

Purposes: Used for cutting delicate soft tissue in confined spaces. Also used for micro dissection of arachnoid bands and adhesions in deep cranial and spinal cases.

Varieties: Straight, curved, or angled blades. Various lengths of arms.

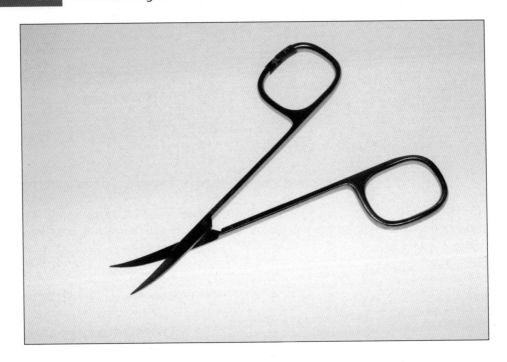

Ins Scissors

Alternative Names: Lexer-Baby, Bonn, Kelly, iris scissors, micro dissecting scissors

Category: Scissors

Purposes: Useful for cutting very fine, delicate tissue, including vessels. Can be used to extend arteriotomies, isolate bypass grafts, etc.

Varieties: Straight or curved blades. Various arm lengths.

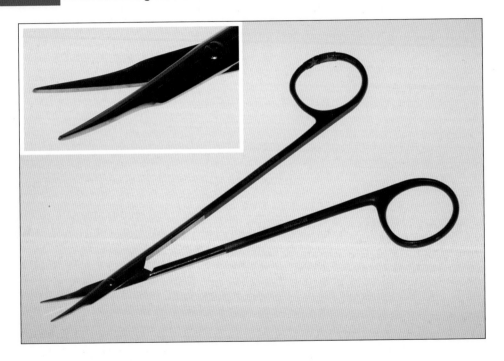

Jameson Tenotomy Scissors

Alternative Names: Jameson-Potts, Jamison-Metz, Jamison-Reynolds, tenotomies, long iris scissors

Category: Scissors

Purposes: Useful for cutting very fine, delicate tissue, including vessels. Can be used to extend arteriotomies, to isolate bypass grafts, in pediatric cases, etc.

Varieties: Straight or curved blades. Various arm lengths.

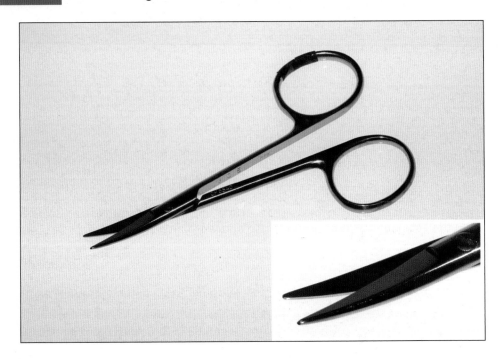

Knapp Iris Scissors

Alternative Names: Lexer-Baby, Bonn, Kelly, iris scissors, micro dissecting scissors

Category: Scissors

Purposes: Useful for cutting very fine, delicate tissue, including vessels. Can be used to extend arteriotomies, to isolate bypass grafts, in pediatric cases, etc.

Varieties: Straight or curved blades. Various arm lengths.

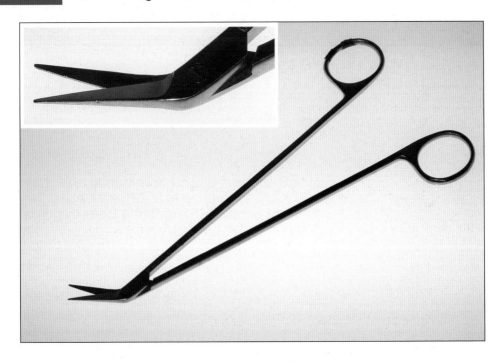

Potts-DeMartel Scissors

Alternative Names: Potts scissors, Potts-Smith, angled scissors, vascular scissors

Category: Scissors

Purposes: Used for cutting vessels, e.g., extending an arteriotomy or venotomy. Can also be used to cut fine, delicate tissue in deep, closed spaces, e.g., to extend dural opening in intramedullary spine or peripheral nerve cases.

Varieties: Variable instrument lengths. Variable blade lengths and angles.

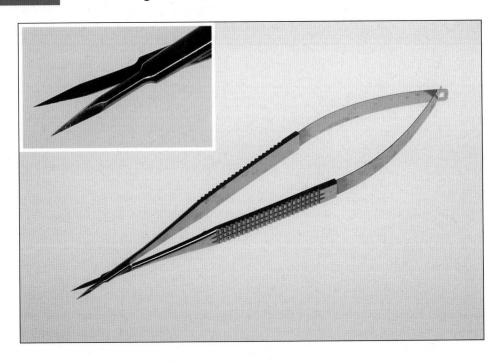

Vannas Micro Scissors

Alternative Names: Hoyes micro scissors, Westcott scissors, micro scissors

Category: Scissors

Purposes: Used for cutting delicate soft tissue in confined spaces. Also used for micro dissection of arachnoid bands and adhesions in deep cranial and spinal cases.

Varieties: Straight, curved, or angled blades. Various lengths of arms.

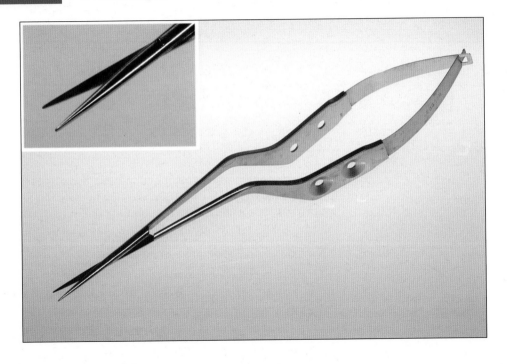

Yasargil Bayonet Scissors

Alternative Names: Bayonet scissors, aneurysm scissors

Category: Scissors

Purposes: Used for cutting delicate soft tissue in confined spaces. Also used for gross removal of large tumors or initial cuts in giant aneurysm sacs.

Varieties: Straight, curved, or angled blades. Various lengths of arms.

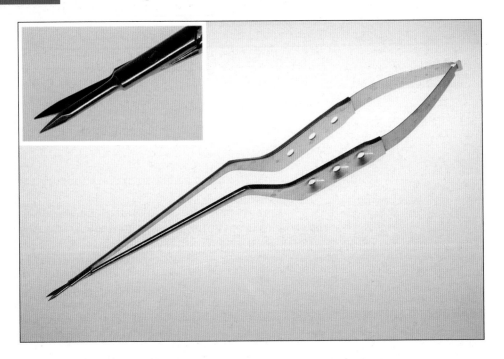

Yasargil Bayonet Micro Scissors

Alternative Names: Micro scissors, bayonet micro scissors

Category: Scissors

Purposes: Used for cutting delicate soft tissue in confined spaces. Also used for micro dissection of arachnoid bands and adhesions in deep cranial and spinal cases.

Varieties: Straight, curved, or angled blades. Various lengths of arms.

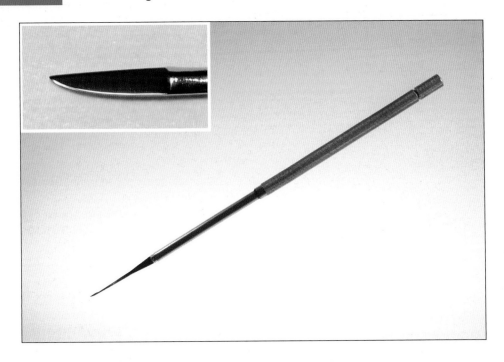

Arachnoid Knife

Alternative Name: Beaver blade

Category: Knives

Purposes: Used to isolate aneurysmal lesion from the parent circulation. Can also be used to ligate bleeding vessels unable to be cauterized, e.g., AVM cases or fistulous lesions, or for temporary occlusion of larger vessels during revascularization procedures, endarterectomies, and tumor resections. For aneurysms, clips can be loaded in various positions, e.g., curve down, angle up, legs up, etc. Newer appliers have adjustable, flexible, or rotating ends, making virtually all clip positions possible. A review of all available systems is beyond the scope of this guide.

Varieties: Infinite. Straight, curved, angled, fenestrated, bayoneted, mini, temporary, and any combination of the above. Several new materials and alloys have been recently introduced. Opening/closing mechanism is also variable. The standard spring compression is demonstrated here. Please see manufacturer's information guide for more specific mechanics of utilized system.

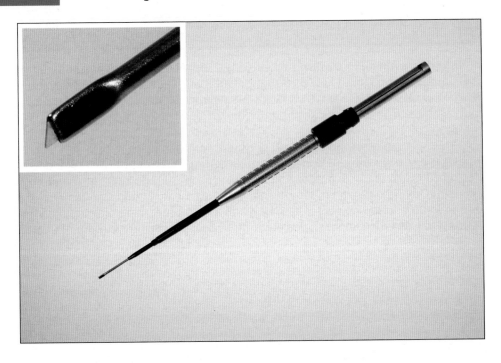

Diamond Knife

Alternative Name: None

Category: Knives

Purposes: Used for fine dissection or cutting of delicate tissues. Useful in dissecting aneurysmal or other vascular lesions and adherent tumors, or in generalized sharp dissection. A sleeve is pulled over the blade for protection, given its delicate nature.

Varieties: Variable types of handles. Triangular or square diamond blades.

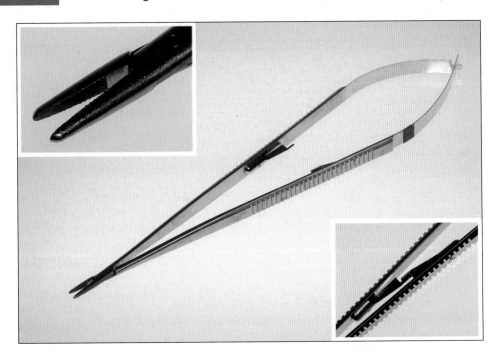

Castroviejo Needle Holder

Alternative Names: Micro needle holder, micro locking needle holder

Category: Needle holders

Purposes: Microsurgical needle holder with locking mechanism reducing pressure required to hold needle. Spring-like opening of jaws when not locked. Used most commonly for microsuturing.

Varieties: Straight or curved jaws. Rounded and flat side arms.

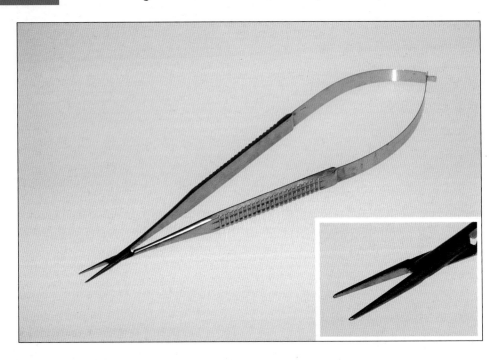

Micro Needle Holder

Alternative Names: Barraquer needle holder, Patton needle holder, Sklar micro needle holder, micro needle driver

Category: Needle holders

Purposes: Non-locking needle holder used for holding and manipulating small needles and suture in confined spaces. Most often used in microvascular, peripheral nerve, and intradural cases.

Varieties: Various lengths of arms. Various sizes of jaws.

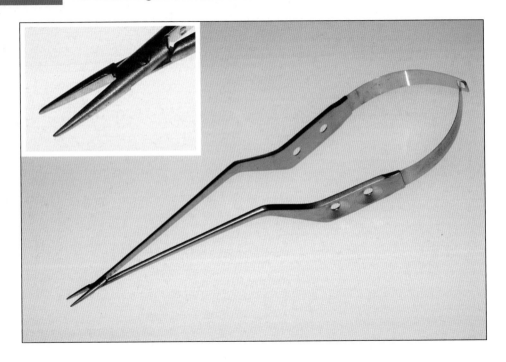

Yasargil Bayonet Needle Holder

Alternative Names: Bayonet needle holder, bayonet micro needle holder

Category: Needle holders

Purposes: Non-locking bayonet needle holder used for holding and manipulating small needles and sutures in confined spaces. Most often used in microvascular, intradural, and peripheral nerve/re-anastomoses cases.

Varieties: Various lengths of arms. Various sizes of jaws.

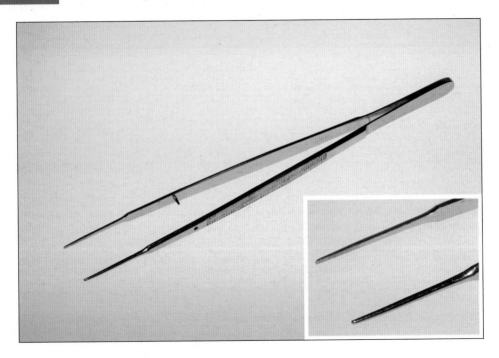

Gerald Forceps without Teeth

Alternative Names: Pickups without teeth, Gerald without, Cushing forceps (incorrect)

Category: Forceps

Purposes: Non-traumatic grasping and holding forceps designed for very delicate tissue or vessels. Can be used to hold vessels or open the vessel lumen. Can also be used for handling tubing and other surgical implants and their cables.

Varieties: None.

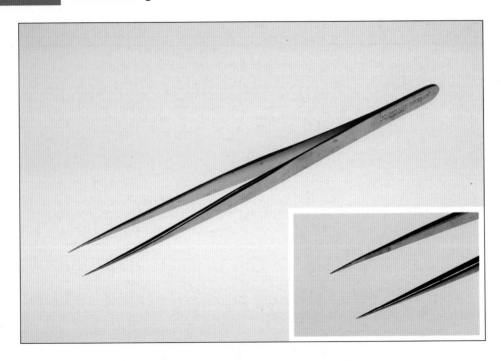

Micro Suture Forceps

Alternative Names: Jewelers, micro forceps

Category: Forceps

Purposes: Used to grasp and manipulate fine, delicate tissue, e.g., nerve or vessels, or as a micro-needle holder. Often used in microvascular, intradural, and peripheral nerve/re-anastomosis procedures.

Varieties: Straight or curved tips. Various lengths of arms.

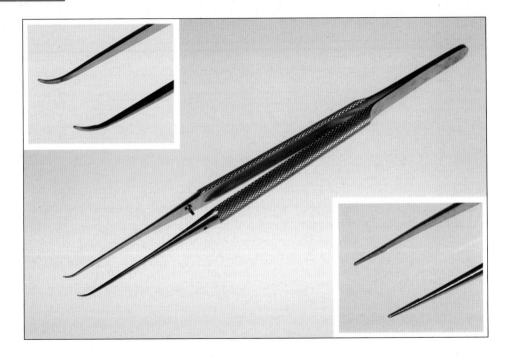

Round Body Forceps

Alternative Names: Round jeweler's forceps, round micro forceps

Category: Forceps

Purposes: Used for grasping and manipulating fine, delicate tissue, e.g., nerve or vessels, or as a micro-needle holder. Often used in microvascular, intradural spine, and peripheral nerve/re-anastomosis procedures. Round shaft allows rotation of instrument.

Varieties: Straight or curved tips. Various lengths of arms.

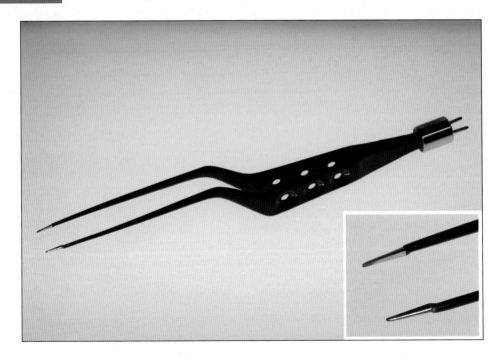

Yasargil Bayonet Bipolar Forceps

Alternative Names: Cushing bipolars, Rhoton forceps, Malis bipolars, bayonet, bipolar forceps, bipolars

Category: Forceps

Purposes: Coagulation of tissue between the tips of the forceps, which must be in close contact to allow current to flow through tissue. Variable current allows highly tailored effectiveness. Can be used as a dissection instrument or for general grasping of delicate tissue.

Varieties: Straight, curved, or angled tips. Insulated tips or not. Irrigating or not. Short and long. Blunt or fine tips.

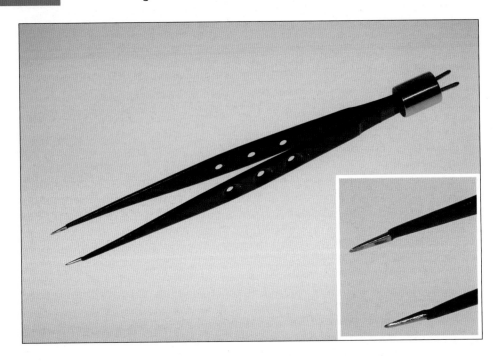

Yasargil Bipolar Forceps Straight

Alternative Names: Straight Cushing bipolars, straight Rhoton forceps, straight Malis bipolars, straight bipolar forceps, straight bipolars

Category: Forceps

Purposes: Coagulation of tissue between the tips of the forceps, which must be in close contact to allow current to flow through tissue. Variable current allows highly tailored effectiveness. Can be used as a dissection instrument or for general grasping of delicate tissue.

Varieties: Insulated tips or not. Short and long. Blunt or fine tips.

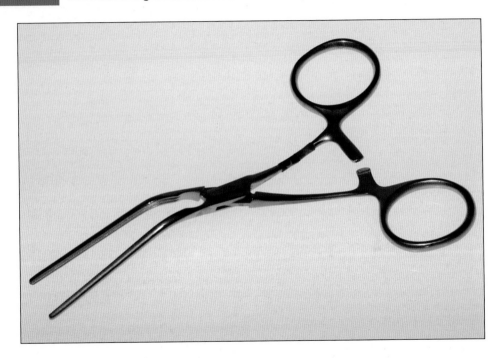

Cooley Clamp

Alternative Names: DeBakey clamp, carotid clamp, bulldog clamp, angled clamp

Category: Clamps

Purposes: Used for temporary occlusion of large blood vessels. Most commonly used for common carotid artery occlusion during endarterectomies, intraoperative internal carotid artery access, etc.

Varieties: None.

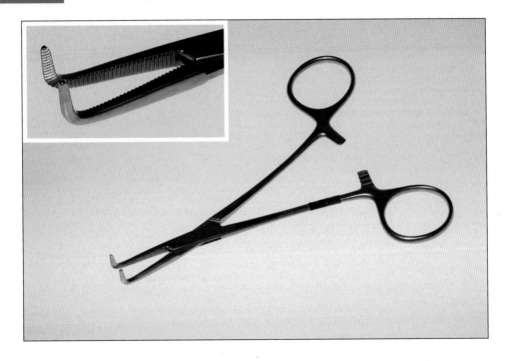

Mixter Right Angle Clamp

Alternative Names: Right angle, right angle hemostat, right angle snap, right angle Adson clamp, right angle Crile clamp

Category: Clamps

Purposes: Used for dissecting and isolating delicate soft tissues, especially around vessels and nerves. Often used to grasp tying sutures to pull them underneath these structures in preparation for ligation. Also used for dissecting tissue underneath or around structures.

Varieties: Variable lengths of arms and handles.

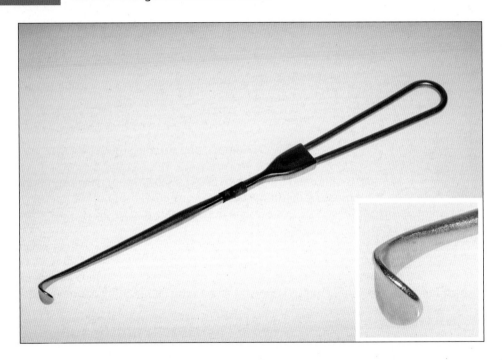

Cushing Vein Retractor

Alternative Names: Vein retractor, Cushing retractor, Sachs retractor

Category: Retractors

Purposes: Retraction, lifting, or isolation of delicate soft tissue and vessels.

Varieties: Solid or fenestrated blade. Variably sized end.

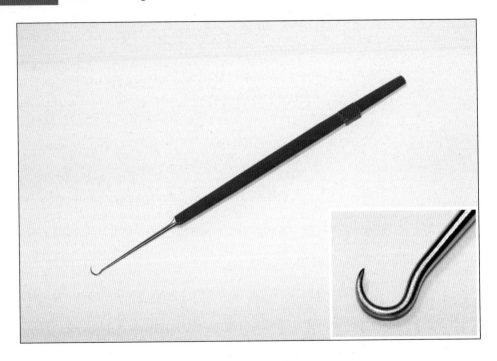

Frazier Dural Retractor

Alternative Names: Dural hook, dural elevator, micro hook, Adson hook, Fisch hook (incorrect)

Category: Retractors

Purposes: Used for retraction and sharp dissection of fine, delicate soft tissue. Most often used to elevate tissues, especially dura. Very sharp and should be handled and exchanged with care.

Varieties: None.

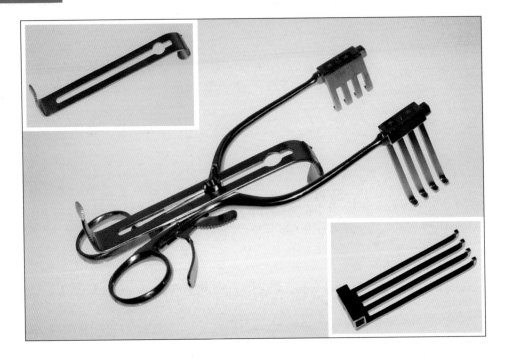

Henly Retractor

Alternative Names: Mayo-Adams retractor, cervical retractor

Category: Retractors

Purposes: Used for retraction of skin and soft tissues to allow for improved visualization. Used most commonly in cervical spine exposures, but can be used in any small exposure.

Varieties: Sharp or blunt blades. Various lengths, widths, and number of teeth on the blades.

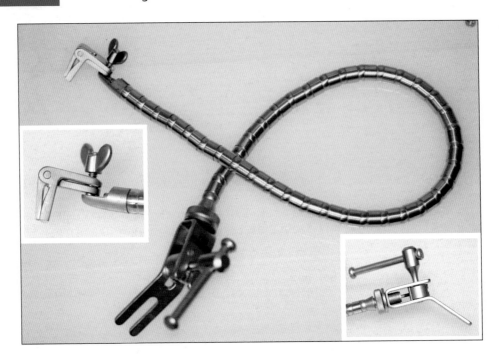

Leyla-Yasargil Retractor Arm

Alternative Names: Fixation base, snake holder, snake charmer

Category: Retractors

Purposes: Fits on the end of the Leyla bar and allows the attachment of one to three flexible arms.

Varieties: Number of attachment sites for flexible arms.

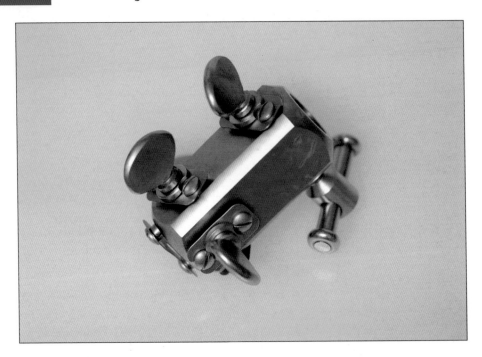

Yasargil Box Connector

Alternative Names: Fixation base, snake holder, snake charmer

Category: Retractors

Purposes: Fits on the end of the Leyla bar and allows the attachment of one to three flexible arms.

Varieties: Number of attachment sites for flexible arms.

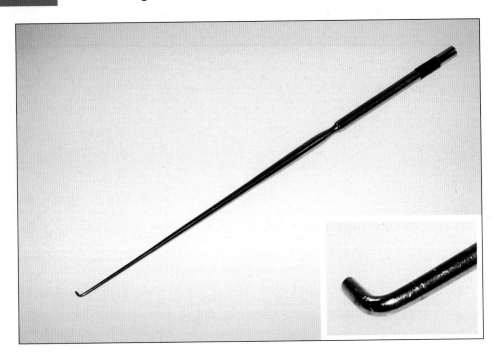

Dandy Nerve Hook

Alternative Names: Nerve hook, Dandy hook

Category: Dissectors

Purposes: Used in exploring, probing, and dissecting fine, delicate soft tissue and nerves. Also used to inspect or find dissection planes underneath and within structures, e.g., thecal sac, disc interspace, etc. The rounded handle allows a rolling, twisting action to sweep tissue away or to work the instrument through tissue planes.

Varieties: None.

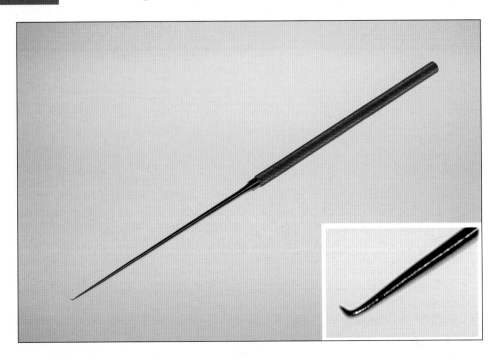

Fisch Sharp Nerve Hook

Alternative Names: Sharp nerve hook, micro hook, Adson hook, Frazier hook (incorrect)

Category: Dissectors

Purposes: Primarily for retraction and sharp dissection of fine, delicate soft tissue. Can also be used to elevate tissues, e.g., dura. Very sharp and should be handled and exchanged with care.

Varieties: Length of tip. Straight or bayonet.

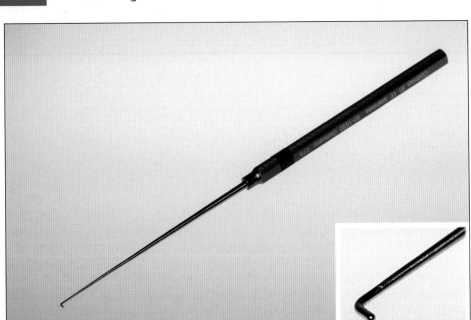

Malis Nerve Hook

Alternative Names: Dandy nerve hook, nerve hook

Category: Dissectors

Purposes: Used for exploring, probing, and dissecting fine, delicate soft tissue and nerves. Used to inspect underneath and within structures. The rounded handle allows a rolling, twisting action to sweep tissue away or to work the instrument between tissue planes.

Varieties: Sharp or blunt tip. Length and angle of tip. Length of shaft.

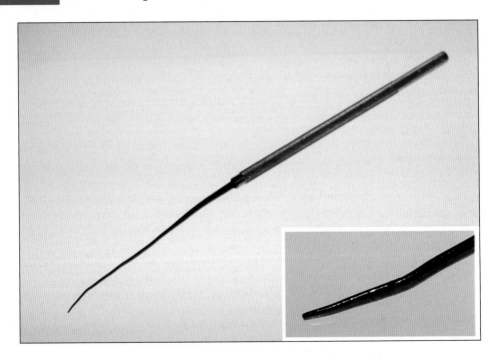

Malleable Micro Dissector

Alternative Names: Dagger, malleable dissector, dissector

Category: Dissectors

Purposes: Used for dissection and mobilization of delicate soft tissue structures, most often used in microsurgical procedures. Often used with vascular lesions, cranio-spinal tumors, skull base procedures, or other entities requiring fine dissection and manipulation.

Varieties: Variable blade width.

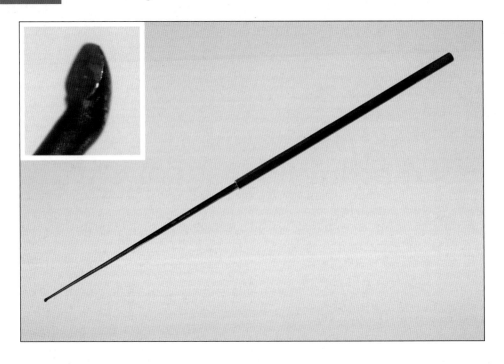

Rhoton #1

Alternative Names: Number 1, small pancake, Janetta dissector, small round dissector

Category: Dissectors

Purposes: Used for microscopic manipulation and dissection of tissues. Sharp dissector edge allows scraping of tissue off other structures, sharp cutting of adherent tissue adhesions, and focal retraction.

Varieties: Straight or angled shaft.

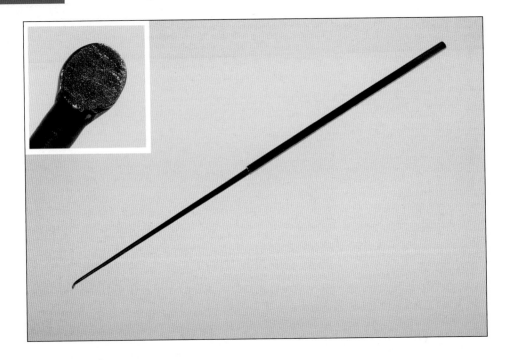

Rhoton #2

Alternative Names: Number 2, medium pancake, pancake, Janetta dissector, medium round dissector

Category: Dissectors

Purposes: Used for microscopic manipulation and dissection of tissues. Sharp dissector edge allows scraping of tissue off other structures, sharp cutting of adherent tissue adhesions, and focal retraction.

Varieties: Straight or angled shaft.

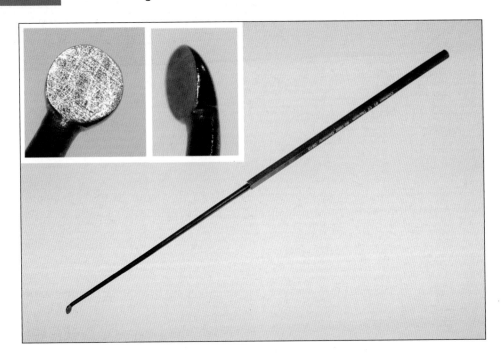

Rhoton #3

Alternative Names: Number 3, large pancake, pancake, Janetta dissector, large round dissector

Category: Dissectors

Purposes: Used for microscopic manipulation and dissection of tissues. Sharp dissector edge allows scraping of tissue off other structures, sharp cutting of adherent tissue adhesions, and focal retraction.

Varieties: Straight or angled shaft.

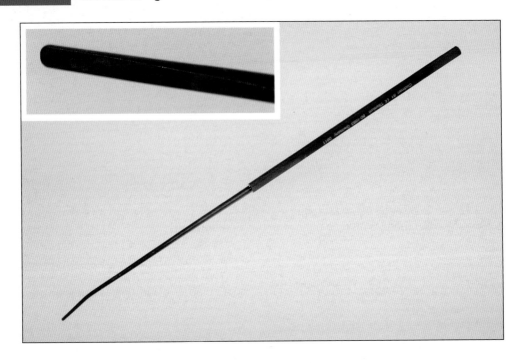

Rhoton #4

Alternative Names: Number 4, small elevator, micro elevator, Janetta elevator

Category: Dissectors

Purposes: Used for microscopic manipulation and dissection of delicate tissues, e.g., nerves, vessels, etc. Also used for blunt dissection and exploration of microscopic tissue planes.

Varieties: Straight or angled shaft.

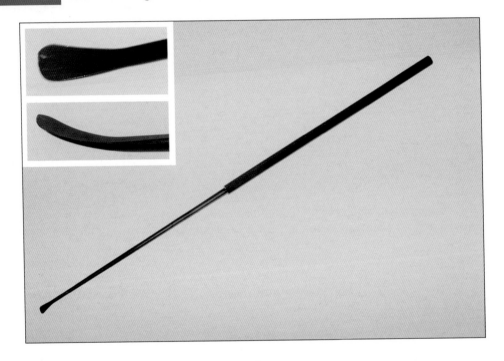

Rhoton #5

Alternative Names: Number 5, large micro elevator, micro elevator, Janetta elevator

Category: Dissectors

Purposes: Used for microscopic manipulation and dissection of delicate tissues, e.g., nerves, vessels, etc. Also used for blunt dissection and exploration of microscopic tissue planes.

Varieties: Straight or angled shaft.

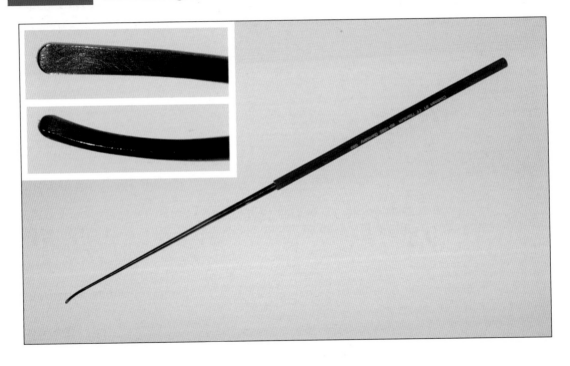

Rhoton #6

Alternative Names: Number 6, micro dissector, Janetta elevator, spatula dissector, micro spatula

Category: Dissectors

Purposes: Used for microscopic manipulation and dissection of delicate tissues, e.g., nerves, vessels, etc. Also used for blunt dissection and exploration of microscopic tissue planes.

Varieties: Straight or angled shaft.

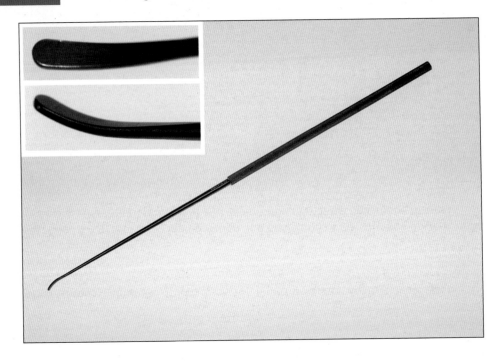

Rhoton #7

Alternative Names: Number 7, micro dissector, Janetta elevator, spatula dissector, micro spatula, medium micro spatula

Category: Dissectors

Purposes: Used for microscopic manipulation and dissection of delicate tissues, e.g., nerves, vessels, etc. Also used for blunt dissection and exploration of microscopic tissue planes.

Varieties: Straight or angled shaft.

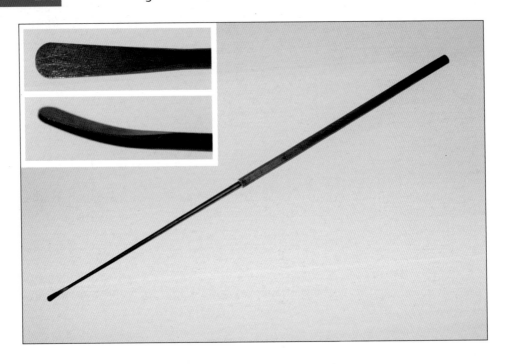

Rhoton #8

Alternative Names: Number 8, micro dissector, Janetta elevator, spatula dissector, micro spatula, large micro spatula

Category: Dissectors

Purposes: Used for microscopic manipulation and dissection of delicate tissues, e.g., nerves, vessels, etc. Also used for blunt dissection and exploration of microscopic tissue planes.

Varieties: Straight or angled shaft.

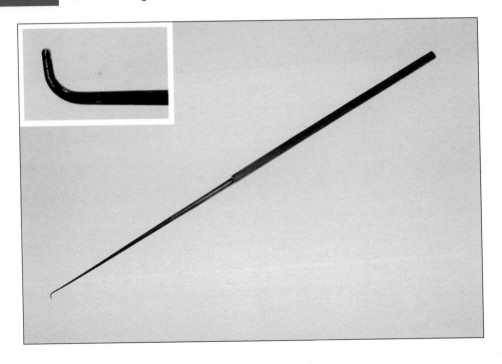

Rhoton #9

Alternative Names: Number 9, micro nerve hook, micro nerve dissector

Category: Dissectors

Purposes: Used for microscopic manipulation and dissection of delicate tissues, e.g., nerves, vessels, etc. Semi-sharp hook allows blunt dissection and exploration of microscopic tissue planes.

Varieties: Straight or angled shaft.

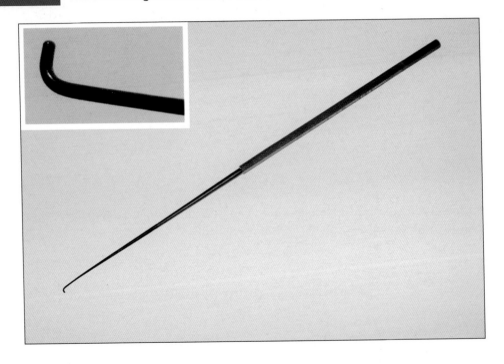

Rhoton #10

Alternative Names: Number 10, micro nerve hook, micro blunt hook, micro nerve dissector

Category: Dissectors

Purposes: Used for microscopic manipulation and dissection of delicate tissues, e.g., nerves, vessels, etc. Blunt hook allows dissection and exploration of microscopic tissue planes.

Varieties: Straight or angled shaft.

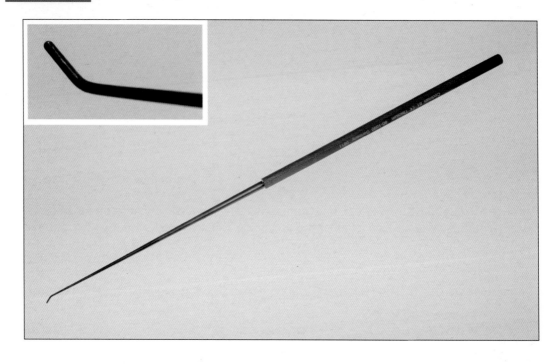

Rhoton #11

Alternative Names: Number 11, micro nerve hook, micro angled hook, micro nerve dissector

Category: Dissectors

Purposes: Used for microscopic manipulation and dissection of delicate tissues, e.g., nerves, vessels, etc. Angled semi-sharp hook allows dissection and exploration of microscopic tissue planes.

Varieties: Straight or angled shaft.

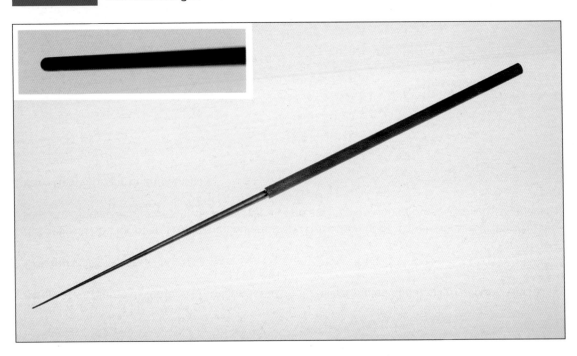

Rhoton #12

Alternative Names: Number 12, micro dissector, micro nerve dissector

Category: Dissectors

Purposes: Used for microscopic manipulation and dissection of delicate tissues, e.g., nerves, vessels, etc. Micro point allows dissection and exploration of microscopic tissue planes.

Varieties: Straight or angled shaft.

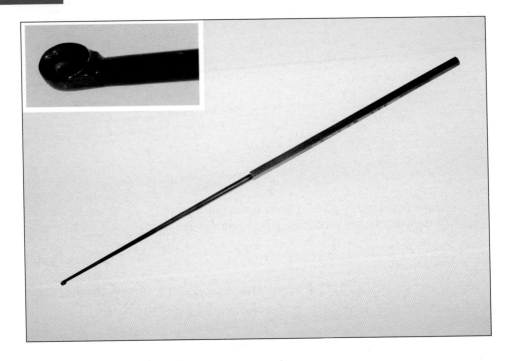

Rhoton #13

Alternative Names: Number 13, micro curette, micro small curette

Category: Dissectors

Purposes: Used for microscopic multipurpose instruments. Scraping tissue off bone, e.g., optic strut, cavernous sinus, foramina, etc., and removing debris. Microcurettes can also be used as dural separators.

Varieties: Straight or angled shaft.

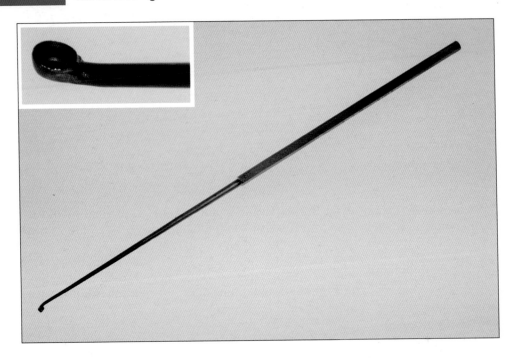

Rhoton #14

Alternative Names: Number 14, micro curette, micro large curette

Category: Dissectors

Purposes: Used for microscopic multipurpose instruments. Scraping tissue off bone, e.g., optic strut, cavernous sinus, foramina, etc., and removing debris. Microcurettes can also be used as dural separators.

Varieties: Straight or angled shaft.

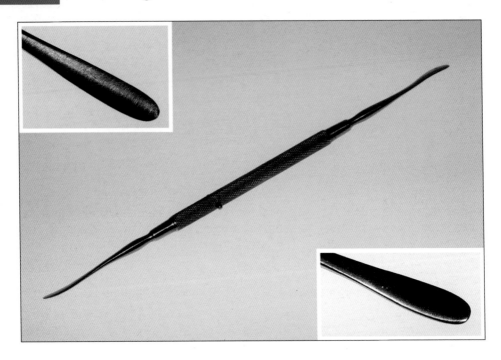

Freer Elevator

Alternative Names: Cottle elevator, Pierce elevator, submucosal elevator

Category: Elevators

Purposes: Multipurpose tool used for separating soft tissue from bone, e.g., nasal septum, skull base, dura, etc.; to dissect vascular plaque in endarterectomies; and even as a protection device when drilling or placing bone wax for hemostasis in narrow spaces.

Varieties: Single- or double-ended. Sharp or blunt blades.

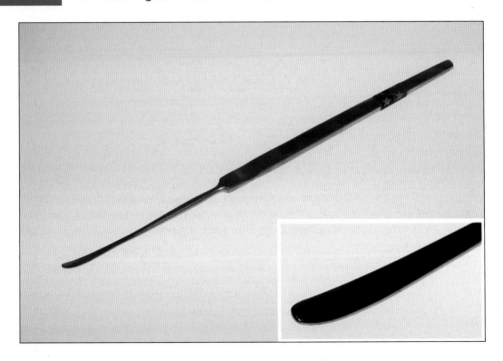

Halle Elevator

Alternative Names: Elevator, tissue elevator, septal elevator (incorrect), Penfield 4 (incorrect)

Category: Elevators

Purposes: Multipurpose tool used in separating soft tissue from bone, e.g., nasal septum, skull base, dura, etc., and even as a protection device when drilling or placing bone wax for hemostasis in narrow spaces.

Varieties: None.

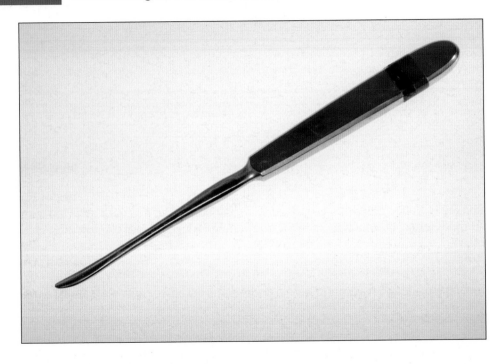

Quervain Elevator

Alternative Names: de Quervain, narrow elevator, periosteal

Category: Elevators

Purposes: Used for scraping tissue from fascia or bone, e.g., periosteum.

Varieties: None.

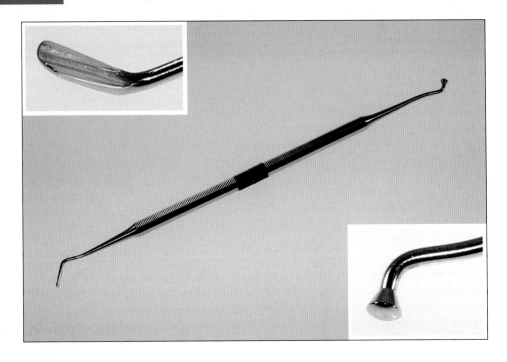

Woodson Dural Separator

Alternative Names: Adson-Woodson (incorrect), dural elevator, groove director, dental instrument

Category: Elevators

Purposes: Double-ended instrument most often used to find tissue planes above dura, e.g., through burr holes, under lamina, etc. Can also be used as a protective instrument when drilling around delicate tissues, e.g., drilling holes for dural tack-up sutures.

Varieties: None.

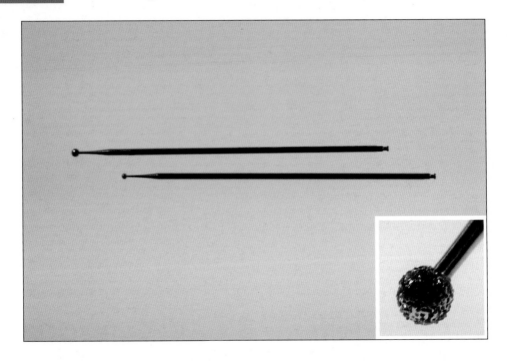

Diamond Burr

Alternative Names: Diamond, coarse diamond bit

Category: Bits

Purposes: Drill bit that allows more precise drilling but requires more time and generates more heat. Often used when drilling around vital structures and in more confined spaces, e.g., clinoidectomies, transverse foramina, etc. Heat generated can be used for hemostasis in more vascularized bone, e.g., sphenoid ridge. Otherwise, copious irrigation is recommended.

Varieties: Fine or coarse bits. Various diameters. Various lengths of the shaft. Various materials.

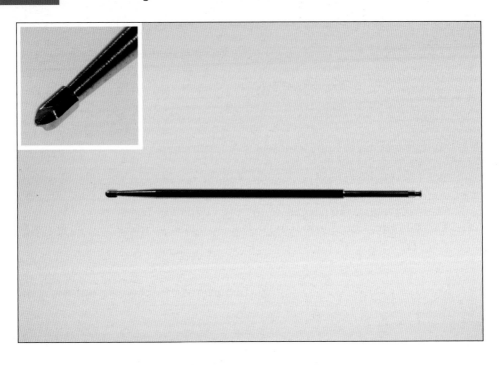

Match Head Drill Bit

Alternative Name: Tapered side cutting, M8, small burr hole bit

Category: Bits

Purposes: Drill bit that allows precision drilling in a side-to-side fashion. The bit is designed not to cut when placed directly on top of structures. Often used for trimming or removing small amounts of undesired bone or thinning out bone above vital structures.

Varieties: Various diameters and lengths of bit.

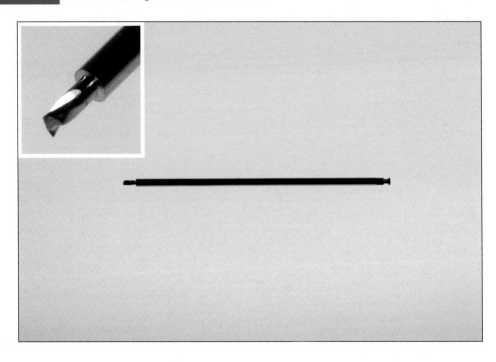

Twist Drill Bit

Alternative Names: Twist drill, screw bit, tap

Category: Bits

Purposes: Tapping holes in bone before screw placement.

Varieties: Various diameters and lengths of bit.

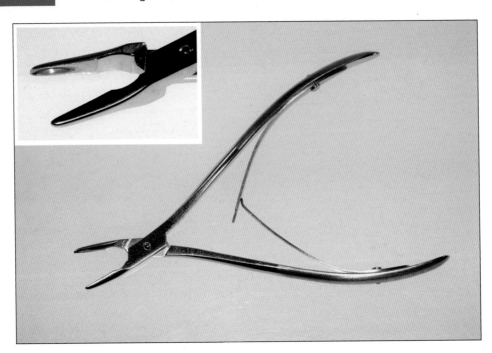

Lempert Rongeur

Alternative Names: Small bone rongeur, Adson rongeur (incorrect), Luer-Friedman, Juers-Lempert, aneurysm rongeur, small bone cutter

Category: Rongeurs

Purposes: Single-action rongeur good for removing small amounts of soft tissue and bone. Often used in confined spaces, e.g., along sphenoid ridge during pterional craniotomies, small amounts of C1 lamina in posterior fossa cases, etc.

Varieties: None.

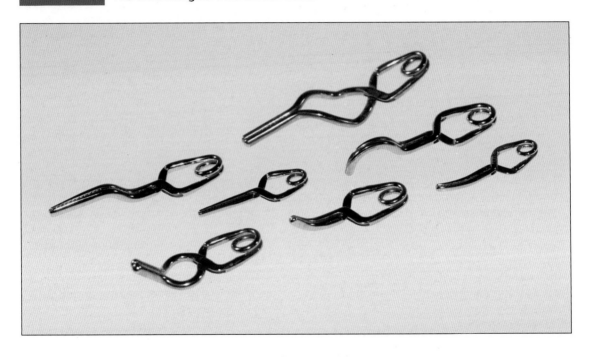

Aneurysm Clips

Alternative Name: None

Category: Specific procedures

Purposes: Used to isolate aneurysmal lesion from the parent circulation. Can also be used to ligate bleeding vessels unable to be cauterized, e.g., AVM cases or fistulous lesions, or for temporary occlusion on larger vessels during revascularization procedures and tumor resections. For aneurysms, clips can be loaded in various positions, e.g., curve down, angle up, legs up, etc. The newest appliers have adjustable, flexible, or rotating jaws, making virtually all clip positions possible.

Varieties: Infinite. Straight, curved, angled, fenestrated, bayoneted, mini, temporary, and any combination above. Several new materials and alloys have been recently introduced. Opening/closing mechanism is also variable. The standard spring compression is shown.

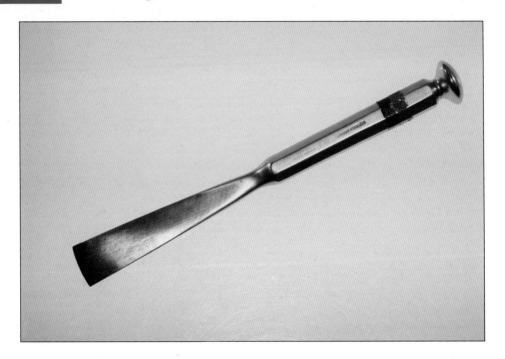

Chisel

Alternative Names: Hibbs chisel, Hoke chisel, osteotome

Category: Specific procedures

Purposes: Used for any modification or sculpting of bone. Selected cranial or spinal cuts, bone graft harvest, and/or molding. Should be used with a mallet.

Varieties: The cutting end can be straight or curved. The lengths of the shaft and width of the cutting blade come in many combinations. The more common are 15 to 25 cm in length and 4 to 25 mm in width.

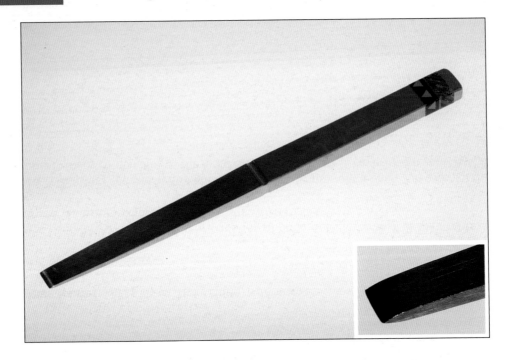

Converse Osteotome

Alternative Names: Osteotome, Lambottle

Category: Specific procedures

Purposes: Any modification or sculpting of bone. Selected cranial or spinal cuts, bone graft harvest, and/or molding. Should be used with a mallet. Usually come as a set.

Varieties: Straight or curved ends. Variable widths of blades.

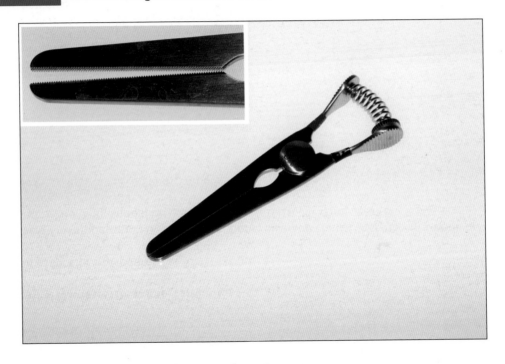

Glover Bulldog Clamp

Alternative Names: Large vessel clamp, Cooley clamp

Category: Specific procedures

Purposes: Occlusion of large vessels, used most frequently in procedures requiring occlusion of large vessels, e.g., endarterectomies, suction decompression for skull base or large ophthalmic/hypophyseal vascular lesions, etc.

Varieties: Various lengths. Smooth or serrated jaws.

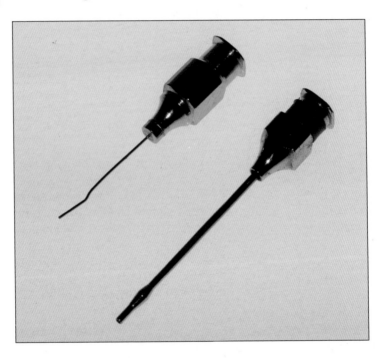

Heparin Needles

Alternative Name: Vessel needles

Category: Specific procedures

Purposes: Attached to syringe to permit the infusion of solutions into vessels, e.g., dilating bypass graft with heparin solution, administration of vasodilators in open-ended vessels, etc.

Varieties: Various sizes.

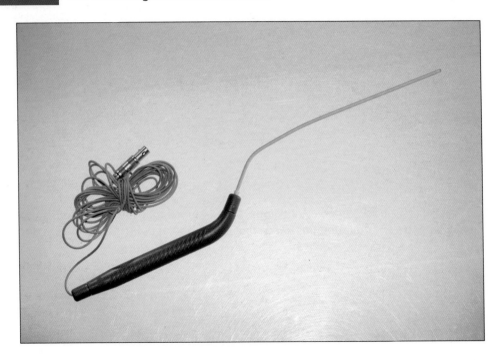

Micro Doppler Probe

Alternative Names: Microvascular Doppler, mini Doppler, bayonet Doppler, vascular Doppler

Category: Specific procedures

Purposes: Allows insonation of the vessels. Often used in determining blood flow after aneurysm clipping, revascularization procedures, fistulae occlusion, and other procedures when the blood flow through particular vessels needs to be determined qualitatively.

Varieties: Bayonet or not. Various diameters of probe tip. Reusable or disposable.

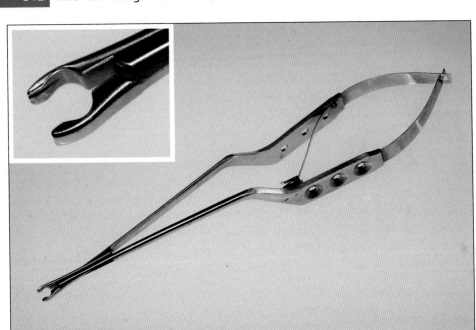

Yasargil Bayonet Aneurysm Clip Applier

Alternative Names: Aneurysm clip applier, large clip applier

Category: Specific procedures

Purposes: Used to secure and apply aneurysm clips. Instrument without locking mechanism is used for clip removal.

Varieties: Straight, curved, or adjustable jaws. With locking mechanism or without.

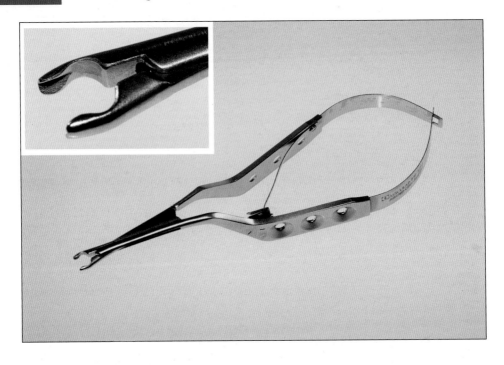

Yasargil Bayonet Aneurysm Mini Clip Applier

Alternative Names: Mini clip applier, small aneurysm clip applier

Category: Specific procedures

Purposes: Used to secure and apply aneurysm clips. Instrument without locking mechanism is used for clip removal.

Varieties: Straight, curved, or adjustable jaws. With locking mechanism or without.

Chapter 6: Spinal Procedures

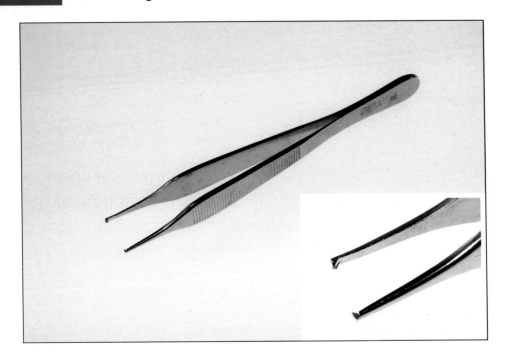

Adson Forceps

Alternative Names: Adson with teeth, Bunny forceps, pickups with teeth, skin forceps, skin pickups

Category: General

Purposes: Used for grasping and holding superficial tissues, especially during closing superficial wounds. Allows precise grabbing of skin edges for improved tissue approximation with minimal tissue injury. Sharp teeth can penetrate fragile tissue, surgical materials (shunt valves, catheters), and gloves.

Varieties: The number of teeth, 1×2 or 2×3. No variety in length.

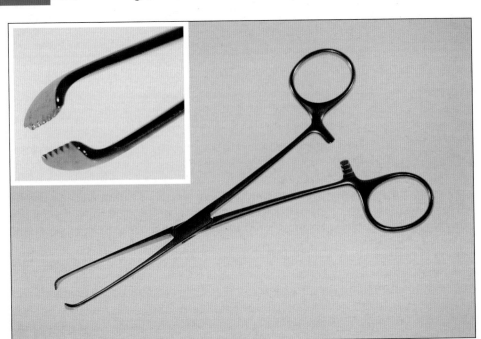

Allis Clamp

Alternative Names: Clamp with teeth, tissue clamp

Category: General

Purposes: Used in securing, lifting, or holding masses or tissue destined for resection, e.g., spinal lipoma, large intracranial meningioma, or fat for fat graft. The interlocking teeth reduce tissue injury. Can also be used for securing cords, cables, and suction tubing to the surgical drapes.

Varieties: The number of teeth, 4×5, 5×6, or 9×10. May be curved or straight and comes in a variety of lengths.

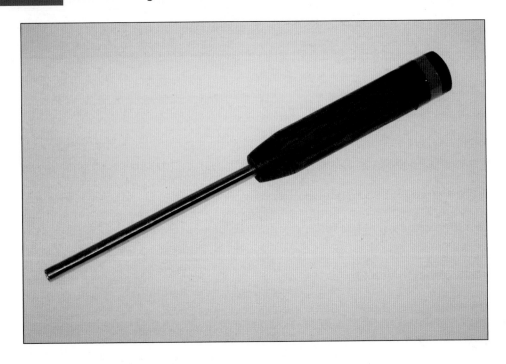

Caspar Screwdriver

Alternative Names: Pin screwdriver, screwdriver

Category: General

Purposes: Allows placement and removal of Caspar pins. Screwdriver end is hollow for placement of Caspar pin into screw guard.

Varieties: Wood or plastic handle.

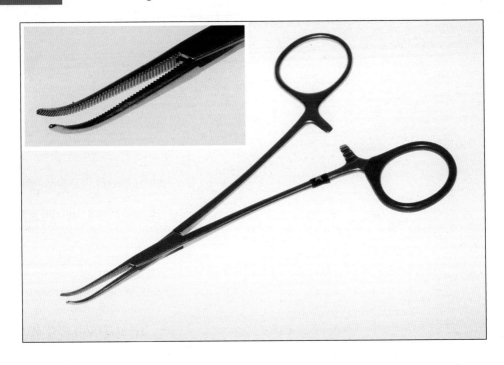

Classic Clamp

Alternative Names: Clamp, Crile clamp, Lahey clamp, Halstead clamp, Adson clamp, Mixter clamp, obtuse clamp, snap, hemostat

Category: General

Purposes: Clamping or occluding vessels or delicate tissue. Used also to dissect tissue planes. Used commonly to grasp and occlude vessels. May be used to pass a suture tie around occluded vessels. Also can be used to secure items to the surgical drape.

Varieties: Straight, curved, and angled. Variable lengths of handles.

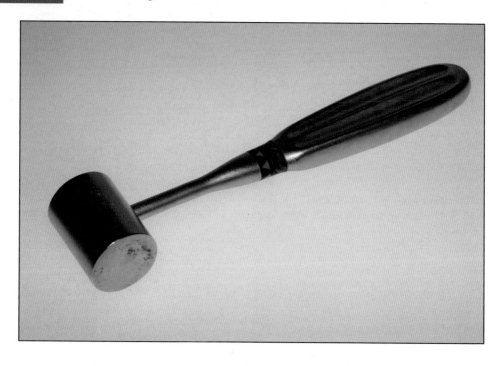

Cottle Mallet

Alternative Names: Mallet, hammer

Category: General

Purposes: Used for application of force, usually on another instrument, e.g., osteotome, bone graft impactor, chisel, etc.

Varieties: Variable weights. Variable material of mallet and handle.

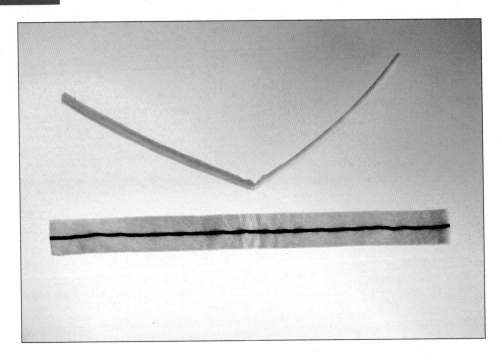

Cotton Patty

Alternative Names: Patty, strip, called out by the measurement of the patty (e.g., half by half), cotton strip or patty

Category: General

Purposes: Multipurpose cotton patties, more commonly used in hemostasis maneuvers involving Gelfoam, Surgicel, or other hemostatic agents. The patty is placed over the agent and the suction draws either blood or fluid, facilitating coagulation. Can be used to apply bone wax atraumatically. Also used as either a wick to draw fluid away or as a protection barrier over vital structures. Many other uses exist. Has a radiopaque strip down the middle.

Varieties: Square and rectangular shapes. Multiple sizes.

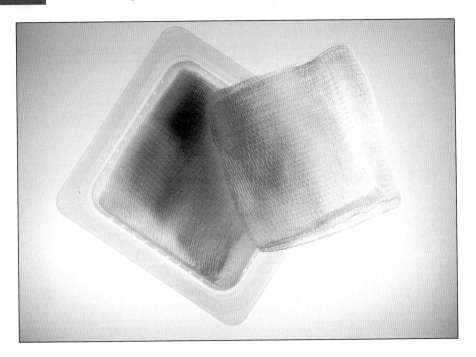

Cotton Sponge

Alternative Names: Ray-tec, sponge, 4×4

Category: General

Purposes: Cotton sheets serving a multitude of purposes, e.g., cleaning, hemostasis, wicking, holding tissue, placement under skin flaps, etc. Filament in sponge allows X-ray detection.

Varieties: Various sizes.

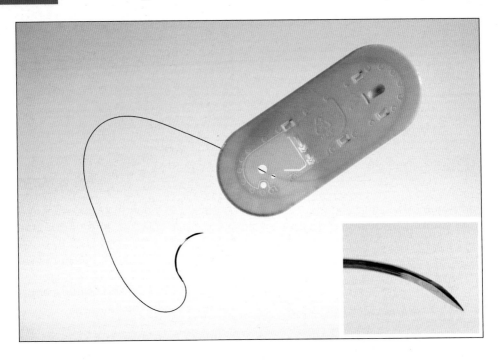

Cutting Suture Needle

Alternative Name: Rarely referred to by their name based on their size

Category: General

Purposes: Triangular-shaped needle tip that cuts through tissue as it is placed through tissue.

Varieties: Straight or curved. Various sizes and diameters of the needle. Various types of suture attached.

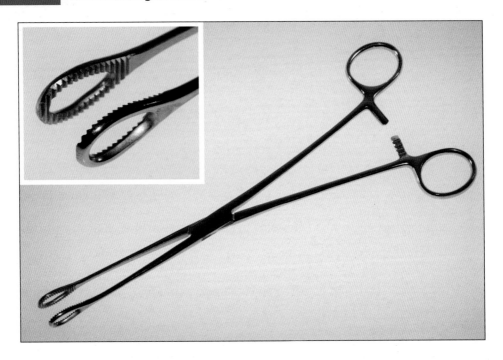

Foerster Sponge Stick

Alternative Names: Sponge stick, ringed forceps, Fletcher sponge stick

Category: General

Purposes: Large forceps good for grasping and holding tissues. Most commonly used with a 4×4 mounted and used for surgical prepping, blunt dissection, and improving visualization by soaking up blood in large wounds.

Varieties: Straight or curved. Variable lengths of arms. Smooth or serrated jaws.

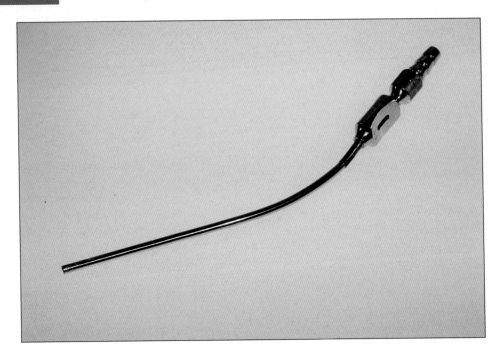

Frazier Suction

Alternative Name: Poppen suction

Category: General

Purposes: Used for suction of fluids in confined spaces. Thumb hole allows on-and-off style of suction. Also used as a retractor, protection device, and blunt dissection tool when removing tumor or brain parenchyma.

Varieties: Straight or angled. Various diameters of tips.

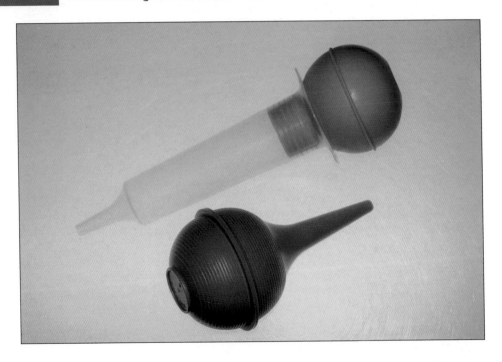

Irrigator

Alternative Names: Asepto, Asepto syringe, bulb syringe, water, big irrigation, flush

Category: General

Purposes: Refillable bulb syringes used for directed irrigation of the surgical site.

Varieties: Multiple sizes and shapes of syringes.

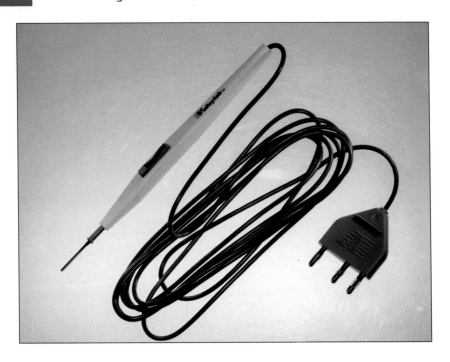

Monopolar

Alternative Names: Bovie, electric knife, cutter, pen knife, cauterizer

Category: General

Purposes: Allows cauterization using high-frequency electrical current through a single electrode that serves as the knife end. The patient's body serves as a ground. Two settings are usually present, one for cutting and the other for cauterization.

Varieties: Universal design. Multiple types of tips, e.g., ring, pinpoint, insulated, etc.

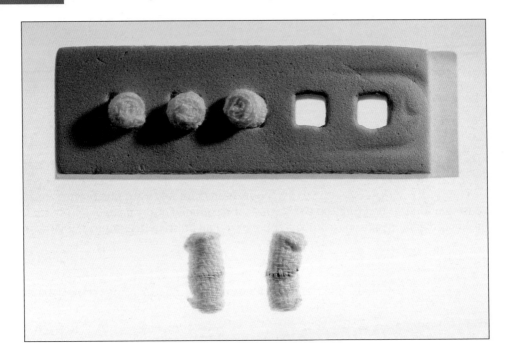

Kittner

Alternative Name: Peanut

Category: General

Purposes: Small rolled-up gauze usually held by a Kelly, Crile, or mosquito clamp and used to dissect tissue bluntly or to clear area for improved visualization. Often used to clean tissue off bone, e.g., prevertebral tissue in ACDFs, lamina for screw placement, etc.

Varieties: Single or multi-packs.

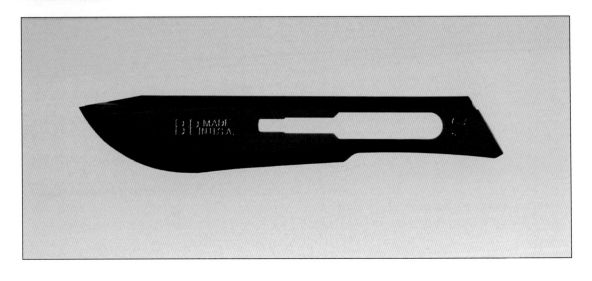

10 Blade

Alternative Name: Skin knife

Category: General

Purposes: Large knife blade often used to make skin incisions.

Varieties: None. Various handle types.

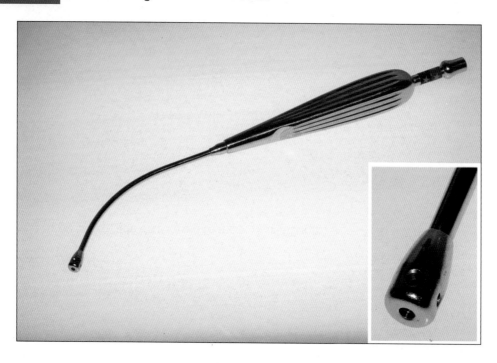

Yankauer Suction

Alternative Name: Tonsil suction tip

Category: General

Purposes: Large-bore suction useful in large surgical exposures. Tip designed to minimize surrounding tissue damage when suctioning.

Varieties: Straight or angled. Protected or non-protected tip. Metal or plastic. Reusable or disposable.

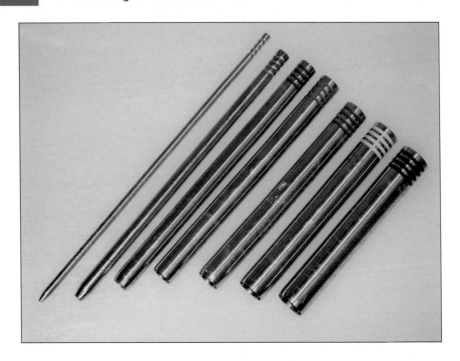

MIS Tubular Retractor Dilators

Alternative Name: None

Category: Dilators

Purposes: Progressive dilators used in minimally invasive spine cases that allow the use of a tubular retraction system. Each dilator is placed over the other and is radiopaque to allow visualization with fluoroscopy.

Varieties: Variable diameter of dilators.

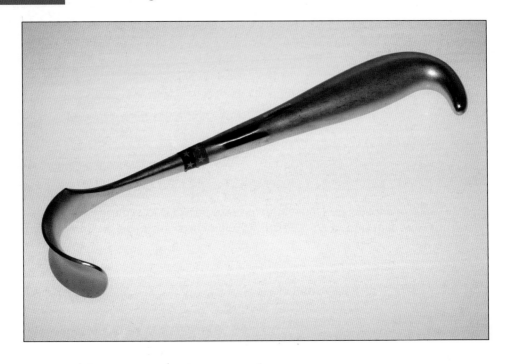

Brewster Retractor

Alternative Names: Tissue retractor, large tissue retractor

Category: Retractors

Purposes: Retraction of surface tissue to allow for improved visualization of the surrounding areas in large wound incisions.

Varieties: None.

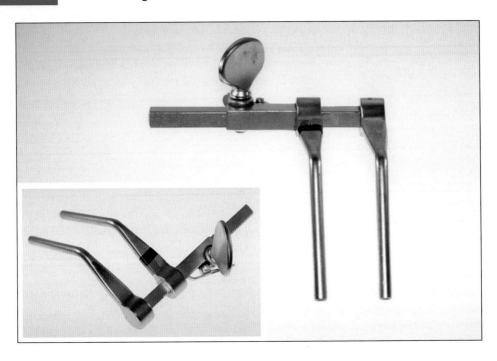

Caspar Retractor

Alternative Names: Distraction pin retractor, pin retractor

Category: Retractors

Purposes: Adjustable and self-retaining retraction system for Caspar pins when performing anterior cervical discectomies.

Varieties: Left- or right-handedness.

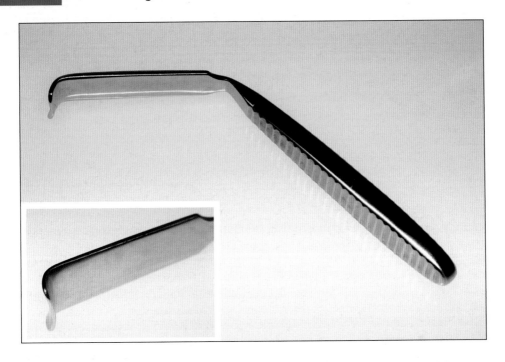

Cloward Hand-Held Retractor

Alternative Names: Hand-held retractor, Cloward retractor

Category: Retractors

Purposes: Used for retraction of surface tissue to allow for improved visualization of the surrounding areas. Often used in anterior cervical spine cases.

Varieties: With and without a lip on the end of the blade.

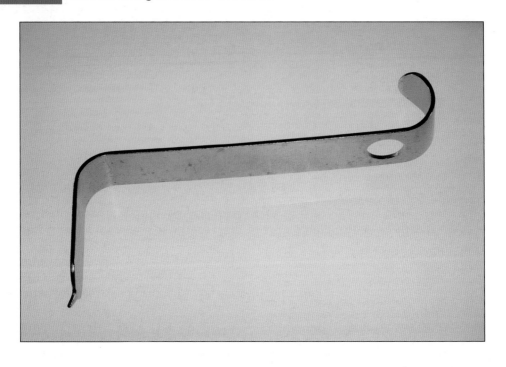

Collis-Taylor Retractor

Alternative Names: Taylor retractor, laminectomy nerve retractor, tissue retractor, large tissue retractor

Category: Retractors

Purposes: Retraction of skin and surface tissue allowing for improved visualization of the surrounding areas. Hook at bottom allows stabilization of retraction against a hard surface, e.g., bone.

Varieties: Lengths of instruments. Small or large blades.

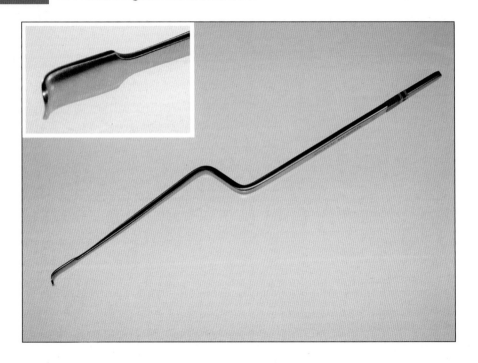

D'Errico Nerve Retractor

Alternative Names: D'Errico, Taylor retractor, laminectomy retractor, tissue retractor, large tissue retractor, nerve root retractor, straight Love retractor, straight Scoville retractor

Category: Retractors

Purposes: Smooth-surfaced, lipped, and crescent-shaped end used for retraction of vital tissue, normally dura or nerve roots during spinal surgery.

Varieties: Straight or angled shaft. Variable blade widths.

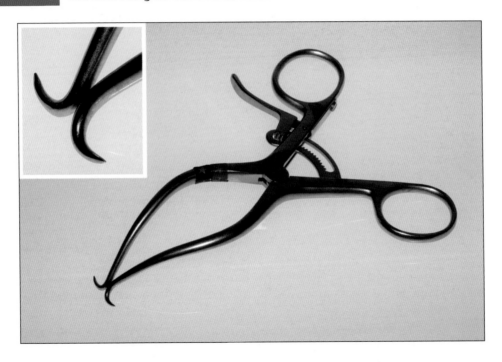

Gelpi Retractor

Alternative Names: Angled Gelpi, short Gelpi

Category: Retractors

Purposes: Used for retraction of surface tissue to allow for improved visualization of the surrounding area. Sharp ends provide point retraction of wound. Used throughout neurosurgical procedures for superficial and deep tissue retraction.

Varieties: Curved and angled ends. Various lengths. Locking and not.

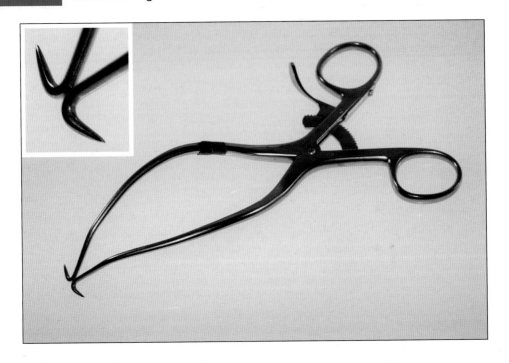

Gelpi Long Retractor

Alternative Names: Angled Gelpi, short Gelpi

Category: Retractors

Purposes: Used for retraction of surface tissue to allow for improved visualization of the surrounding area. Sharp ends provide point retraction of wound. Used throughout neurosurgical procedures for superficial and deep tissue retraction.

Varieties: Curved and angled ends. Various lengths. Locking and not.

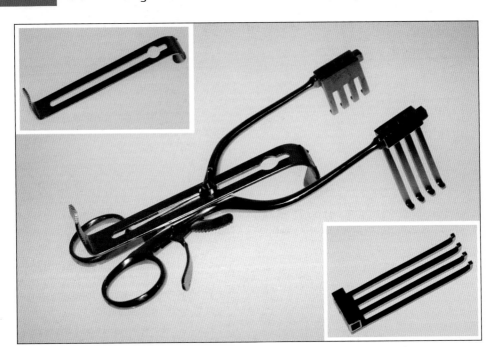

Henly Retractor

Alternative Names: Mayo-Adams retractor, cervical retractor

Category: Retractors

Purposes: Used for retraction of skin and soft tissues to allow for improved visualization. Used most commonly in cervical spine exposures, but can be used in any small exposure.

Varieties: Sharp or blunt blades. Various lengths, widths, and number of teeth on the blades.

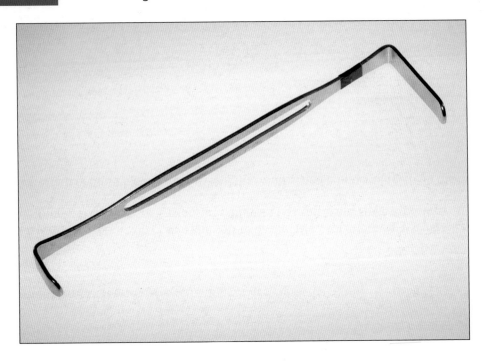

Army-Navy Retractor

Alternative Names: US, Army, US Army, or Navy retractor

Category: Retractors

Purposes: Maintaining retraction in small wounds. Alternatively, these retractors can be used to push tissue out of the way as well. Good for anterior fat harvest, initial parts of MIS (posterior and lateral) cases, and functional implant cases.

Varieties: None.

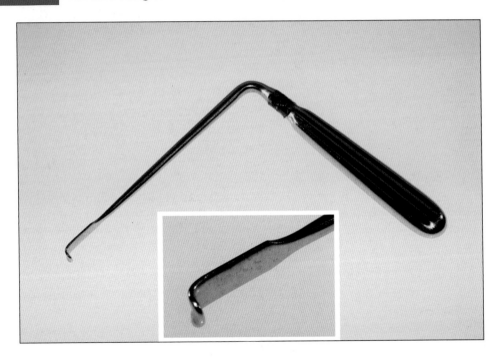

Love Nerve Root Retractor

Alternative Names: Love retractor, angled Scoville retractor, D'Errico (incorrect), Taylor retractor, laminectomy nerve retractor, nerve root retractor

Category: Retractors

Purposes: Smooth-surfaced, lipped, and crescent-shaped end used for retraction of vital tissue, normally dura or nerve roots during spinal surgery.

Varieties: Straight or angled shaft. Variable blade widths. Plastic, metal, or wood handles.

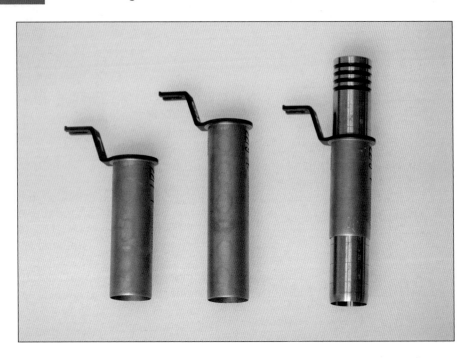

MIS Tubular Retractors

Alternative Name: MIS retractor

Category: Retractors

Purposes: Most commonly used for minimally invasive spine procedures; however, there are some uses in the brain for retractors with smaller diameters. The tube is connected to a stabilizing arm. Some systems have light systems that can be attached. Also, some systems have tubes that can open up further, increasing the exposure.

Varieties: Multiple diameters and lengths. Adjustable and non-adjustable ends. Lighted and non-lighted.

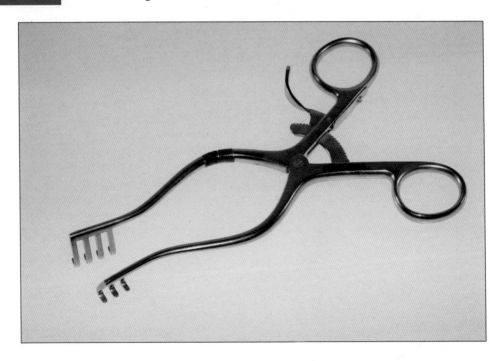

Weitlaner Retractor

Alternative Names: D'Errico-Adson, Mollison, cerebellar, curved cerebellar

Category: Retractors

Purposes: Self-retaining retraction of skin and soft tissue. One of the most common retractors used in neurosurgery.

Varieties: Sharp or blunt teeth. Single or multi-toothed jaws.

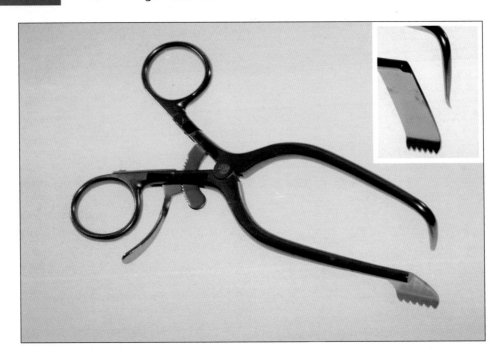

Williams Discectomy Retractor

Alternative Names: Meyerding retractor (incorrect), hemilam retractor, laminectomy retractor

Category: Retractors

Purposes: Deep self-retaining retractor for use when a unilateral lamina is being removed.

Varieties: Right or left orientation (side of the blade).

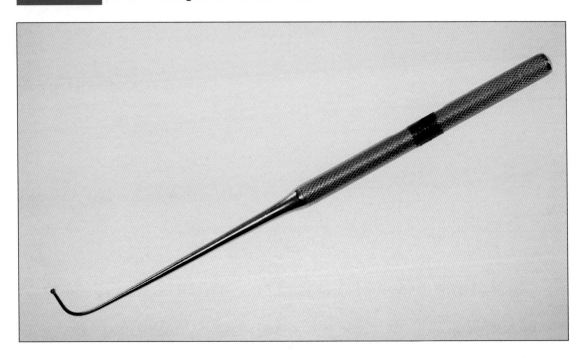

Ball Tip Dissector

Alternative Names: Ball tip probe, ball-tipped nerve hook

Category: Dissectors

Purposes: Used for non-traumatically manipulating tissues including nerves, exploring underneath or within spaces including sub-thecal sac and disc interspaces, and releasing adherent soft tissue.

Varieties: Straight, curved, or angled end. Bayoneted and variable lengths of the shaft.

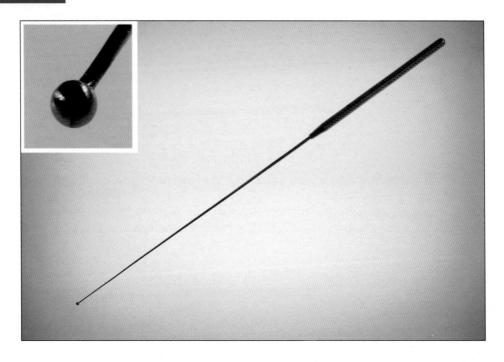

Ball Tip Probe

Alternative Names: Pedicle probe, ball probe, hole probe

Category: Dissectors

Purposes: Used to assess the integrity of the walls in deep bony holes, most often used after drilling and/or tapping pedicle screw pathways. Can also be used to feel the annulus on the other side after discectomy.

Varieties: Various lengths of shaft. With and without rulers.

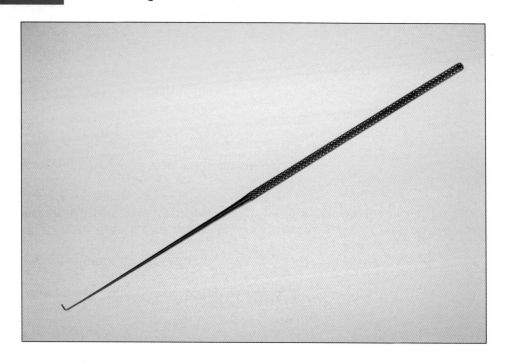

Krayenbuhl Ball Tip Hook

Alternative Names: Ball tip nerve hook, nerve hook

Category: Dissectors

Purposes: Exploring, probing and dissecting fine delicate soft tissue and nerves, most often used to inspect underneath and within structures. The rounded handle allows a rolling, twisting action to sweep tissue away or to work the instrument between tissue planes.

Varieties: Length and angle of tip. Length of shaft.

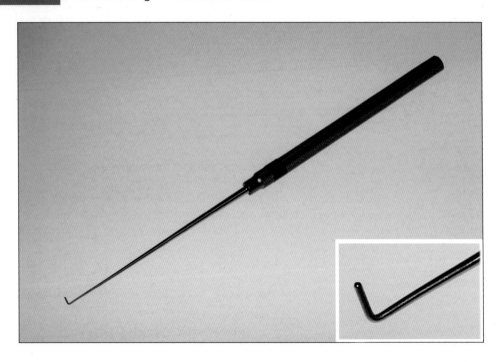

Large Nerve Hook

Alternative Names: Dandy nerve hook, nerve hook

Category: Dissectors

Purposes: Exploring, probing and dissecting fine, delicate soft tissue and nerves, most often used to inspect underneath and within structures. The rounded handle allows a rolling, twisting action to sweep tissue away or to work the instrument between tissue planes.

Varieties: Sharp or blunt tip. Length and angle of tip. Length of shaft.

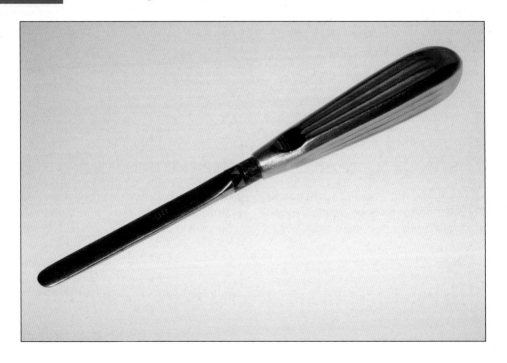

Boles Elevator

Alternative Names: Periosteal, Langenbeck elevator (incorrect), Cobb elevator (incorrect)

Category: Elevators

Purposes: Scraping tissue off fascia and bone, e.g., periosteum. Can also be used to retract or protect soft tissue when drilling through bone (dural tack-up sutures during craniotomy).

Varieties: Sharp/blunt or narrow/wide ends. Curved or straight. Variable length of shaft.

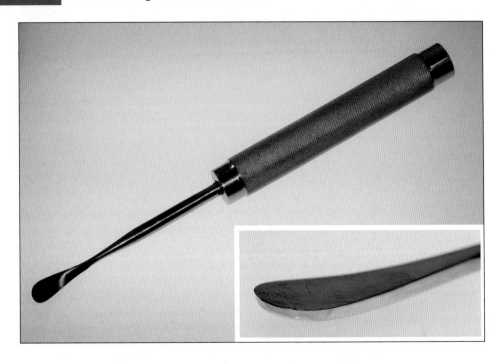

Cobb Elevator

Alternative Names: Periosteal, Langenbeck elevator (incorrect)

Category: Elevators

Purposes: Used in scraping muscle, soft tissue, and periosteum off bone. Can also be used to retract in deep spaces or protect soft tissue when drilling through or on bone. Most often used in posterior spine cases when dissecting muscle and soft tissue around the spinous processes and lamina.

Varieties: Lengths of shaft and size of handle. Variable size of curved end. Wood, plastic, or metal handles.

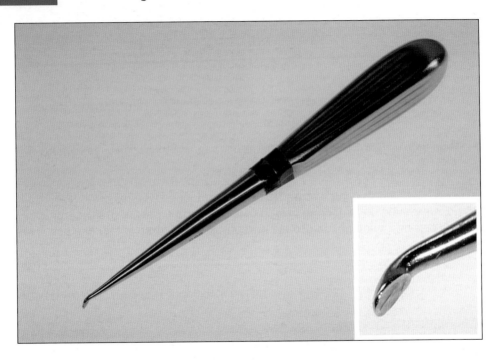

Spinal Fusion Curette

Alternative Names: Brun, bone, oval, round, straight/curved curette

Category: Curettes

Purposes: Multipurpose instrument used for scraping tissue off bone (lateral recess and ligament), sculpting/breaking small areas of bone (optic strut), debriding tissue, or harvesting bone.

Varieties: Straight or angled varieties. The angles can be right, left, upgoing, downgoing, etc. Multiple sizes for cutting end. Can be open or cupped. Various lengths of shaft.

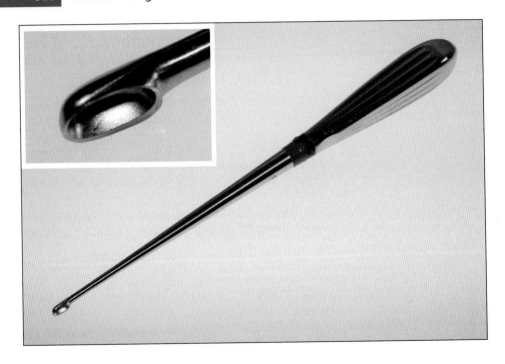

Straight Spinal Fusion Curette

Alternative Names: Brun, bone, oval, round, straight/curved curette

Category: Curettes

Purposes: Multipurpose instrument used for scraping tissue off bone (lateral recess and ligament), sculpting/breaking small areas of bone (optic strut), debriding tissue, or harvesting bone.

Varieties: Straight or angled varieties. The angles can be right, left, upgoing, downgoing, etc. Multiple sizes for cutting end. Can be open or cupped. Various lengths of shaft.

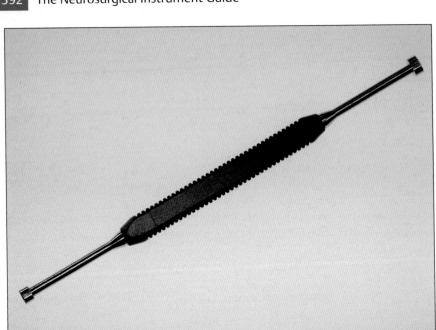

Bone Impactor

Alternative Names: Tamp, impactor

Category: Impactors

Purposes: Impaction of bone graft or other structure, e.g., cage, into place. Used with a mallet.

Varieties: Various diameters of ends. Various lengths. Smooth or sharp end. Metal, plastic or wood handles.

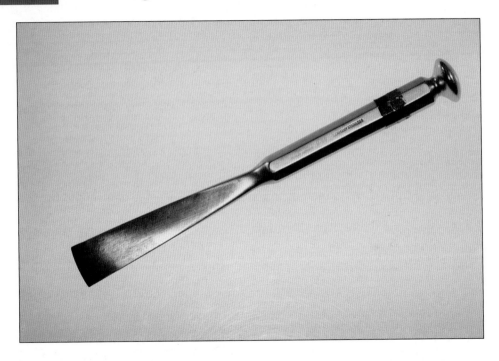

Chisel

Alternative Names: Hibbs chisel, Hoke chisel, osteotome

Category: Impactors

Purposes: Used for any modification or sculpting of bone. Selected cranial or spinal cuts, bone graft harvest, and/or molding. Should be used with a mallet.

Varieties: The cutting end can be straight or curved. The length of the shaft and width of the cutting blade come in many combinations. The more common are 15 to 25 cm in length and 4 to 25 mm in width.

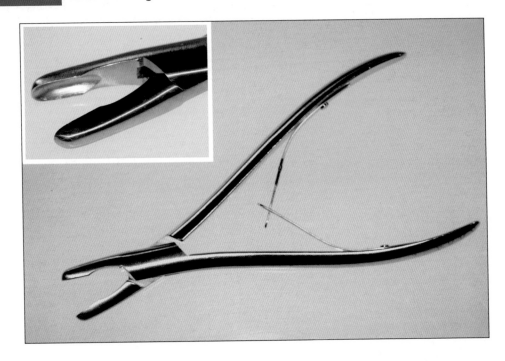

Adson Rongeur

Alternative Names: Bone rongeur, Juers-Lempert or Lempert rongeur (although incorrect), aneurysm rongeur or bone cutter

Category: Rongeurs

Purposes: Removal of bone and soft tissue, often used for removing temporal squamous bone, sphenoid wing, and occipital bone.

Varieties: None.

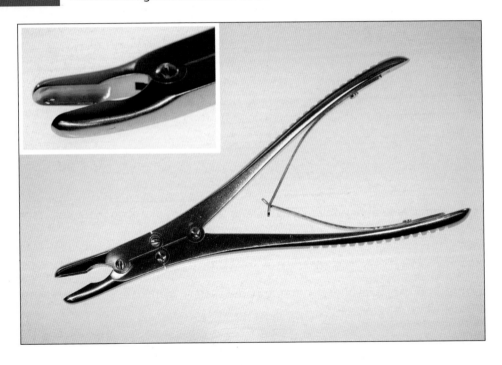

Cushing Rongeur

Alternative Names: Bone rongeur, Adson rongeur, Juers-Lempert or Lempert rongeur (incorrect), aneurysm rongeur (incorrect), small bone cutter

Category: Rongeurs

Purposes: Single-action rongeur good for removing bone and soft tissue. Often used for removing temporal squamous bone, sphenoid wing, and occipital bone. Can also be used in shallow spine cases to remove soft tissue from spinous processes or lamina.

Varieties: None.

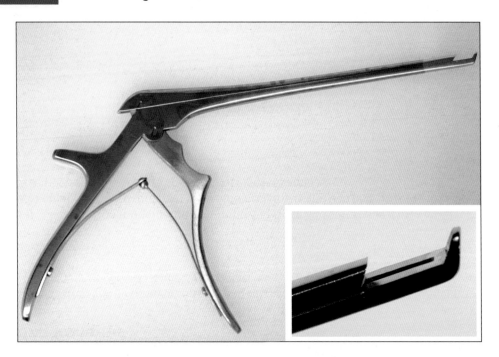

Kerrison Rongeur

Alternative Names: Ruggles, punch, spine rongeur, up or down biting rongeur

Category: Rongeurs

Purposes: Allows precise bone removal by guillotine cutting of small pieces of bone and soft tissue, e.g., ligaments. Foot plate allows stabilization or non-traumatic placement of instrument over vital tissue.

Varieties: Up or down biting. 40°, 45°, or 90° angled tip. Various widths of biting jaw. Coated or non-coated.

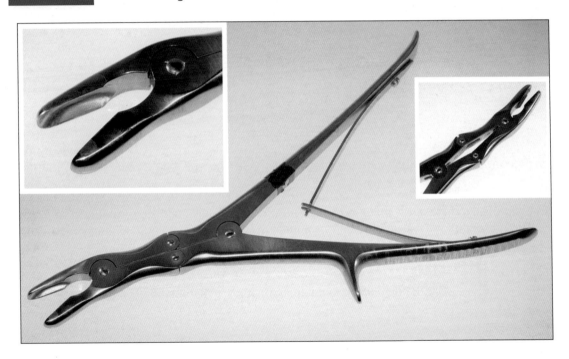

Leksell Stille Rongeur

Alternative Names: Leksell, double-action, large rongeur, Beyer rongeur (incorrect), Luer-Echlin rongeur (incorrect), Sklar-Ruskin rongeur (incorrect), Adson rongeur (incorrect)

Category: Rongeurs

Purposes: Double-action bone rongeur used for removal of bone and soft tissue. Often used for removing temporal squamous bone, sphenoid wing, spinous processes, lamina, osteophytes, and shaping bone flaps. Double action allows more force to be applied to bone.

Varieties: Straight or curved jaws. Variable width of jaws.

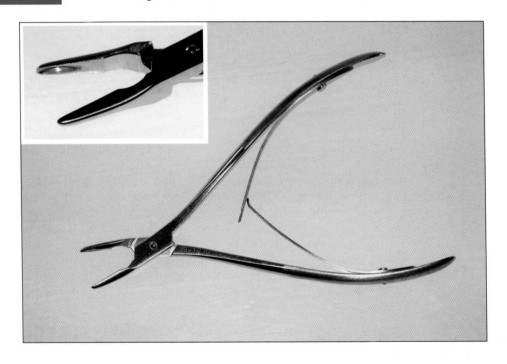

Lempert Rongeur

Alternative Names: Small bone rongeur, Adson rongeur (incorrect), Luer-Friedman, Juers-Lempert, aneurysm rongeur, small bone cutter

Category: Rongeurs

Purposes: Single-action rongeur good for removing small amounts of soft tissue and bone. Often used in confined spaces, e.g., along sphenoid ridge during pterional craniotomies, small amounts of C1 lamina in posterior fossa cases, etc.

Varieties: None.

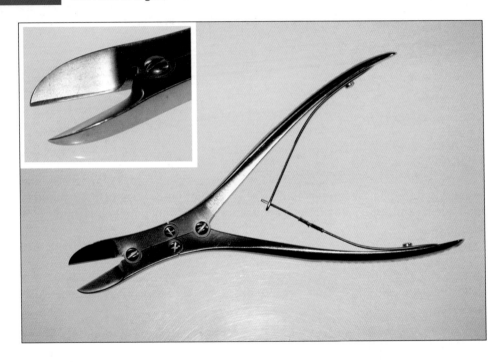

Ruskin-Liston Bone Cutter

Alternative Names: Liston bone cutters, Ruskin cutter, rib shears

Category: Rongeurs

Purposes: Double-action bone cutter used for cutting large pieces of bone, most commonly in spine procedures. Double action allows more force to be applied to bone.

Varieties: Straight or angled blades.

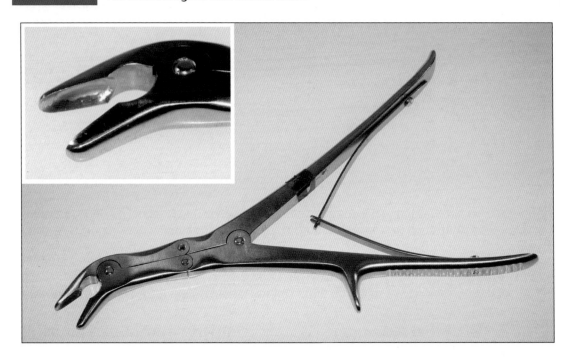

Stille Rongeur

Alternative Names: Duckbill, Sklar-Stille rongeur, Leksell (incorrect), double-action, Beyer rongeur (incorrect), Sklar-Ruskin rongeur (incorrect), Adson rongeur (incorrect)

Category: Rongeurs

Purposes: Double-action bone rongeur used for removal of bone and soft tissue. Often used for removing temporal squamous bone, sphenoid wing, spinous processes, lamina, and osteophytes, and for shaping bone flaps. Double action allows more force to be applied to bone. More narrow jaws allow bone biting in more confined spaces.

Varieties: None.

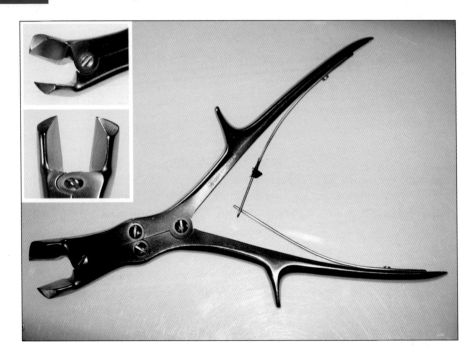

Stille-Horsley Bone Cutter

Alternative Names: Angled Liston (incorrect), angled Ruskin (incorrect), spinous process cutter, big bone cutter

Category: Rongeurs

Purposes: Double-action bone cutter used for cutting large pieces of bone, most commonly in spine procedures. Double action allows more force to be applied to bone. Angled jaws provide good instrument for cuts through the base of the spinous processes.

Varieties: None.

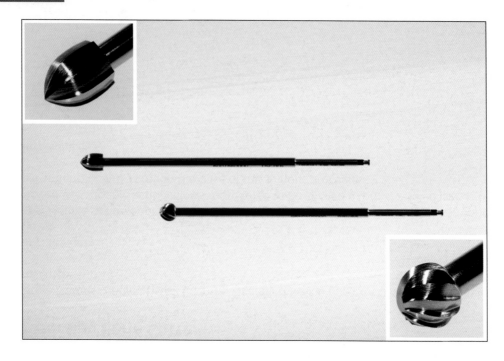

Cutting Drill Bits

Alternative Names: Fluted ball, acorn, round cutter

Category: Drill bits

Purposes: Allow removal of large amounts of bone in a short amount of time through coarse drilling. Can also be used to thin out bone in preparing for punch removal. Caution should be used around delicate structures as these drill bits have no protective features when they come into contact with tissue.

Varieties: Various sizes and shapes of drill bits.

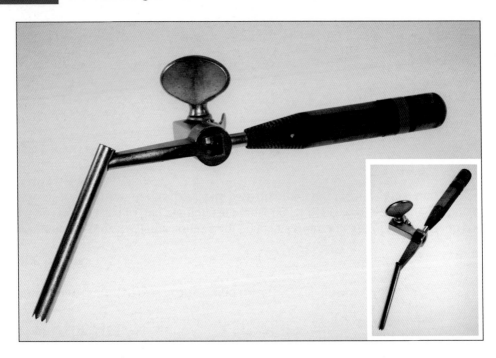

Caspar Drill Guide

Alternative Names: Drill guide, distraction pin drill guide, distraction pin guide

Category: Drill guides

Purposes: Drill guide for placement of distraction pins, often used in anterior cervical spine approaches. Toothed guide allows stable placement on vertebral body. Allows for connection to Caspar pin holder for more precise placement of second Caspar pin.

Varieties: Left- or right-handedness. Wood or plastic handle.

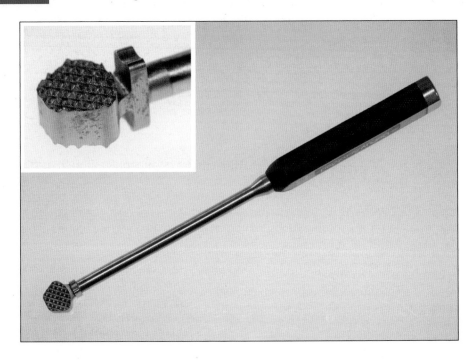

Disc Space Rasper

Alternative Names: Rasp, disc rasp, space filer

Category: Spine fusion instrumentation

Purposes: Preparation of disc space for placement of graft by clearing residual disc material from endplates.

Varieties: Variable heights, widths, and angulation of rasper.

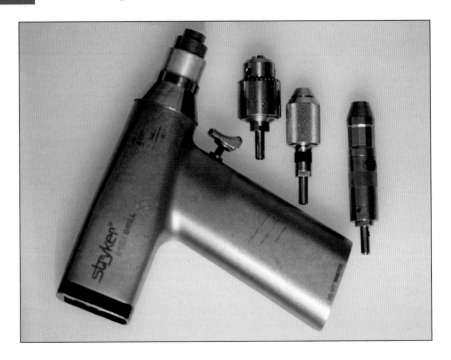

Hand-Held Drill

Alternative Name: None

Category: Spine fusion instrumentation

Purposes: Multipurpose drill, used most often in spine procedures for tapping screw holes or preparing bone grafts.

Varieties: Various drill bit holder attachments.

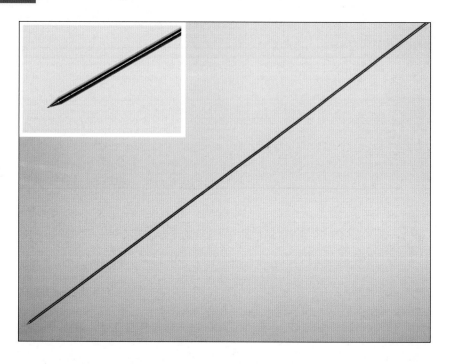

K-wire

Alternative Name: None

Category: Spine fusion instrumentation

Purposes: Long metal wire used for localizing and maintaining position of desired screw trajectories during MIS procedures.

Varieties: Sharp or blunt tip.

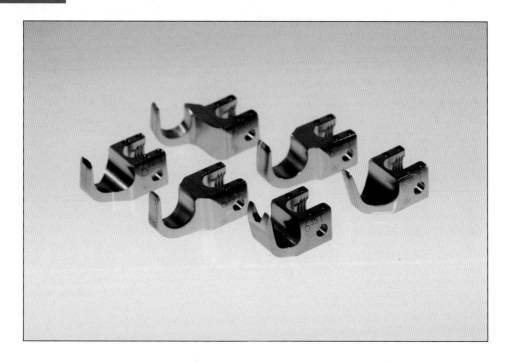

Laminar Hooks

Alternative Name: Hook

Category: Spine fusion instrumentation

Purposes: Used most often for vertebral levels with pedicles too small for screw placement or for a mechanistic bolster.

Varieties: Various orientations and sizes of hooks.

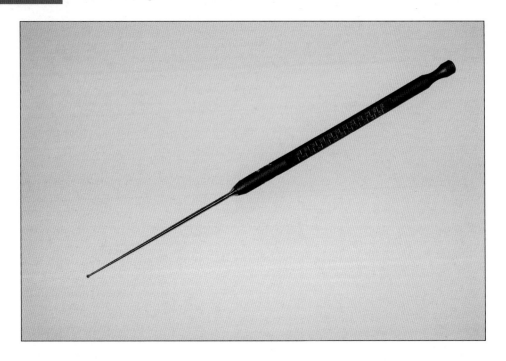

Pedicle Depth Probe

Alternative Names: Pedicle probe, ball probe, hole probe

Category: Spine fusion instrumentation

Purposes: Used to assess the integrity of the surrounding bony walls and measure the depth in deep bony holes. Most often used after drilling and/or tapping pedicle screw pathways. Aids with assessing desired screw length.

Varieties: Various lengths of shaft. With and without rulers.

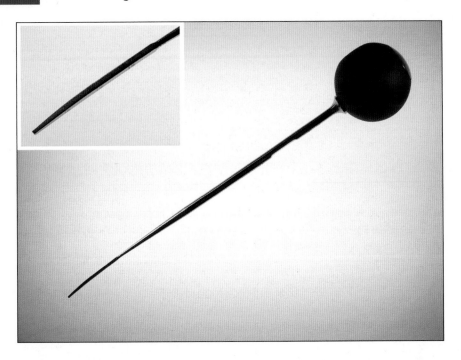

Pedicle Finding Awl

Alternative Names: Gearshift, pedicle awl

Category: Spine fusion instrumentation

Purposes: Used for establishing initial bony pathway through pedicle and vertebral body for screw placement. Tapered end travels through trabecular bone. Curved end can assess for cortical bony walls as it traverses the trabecular bone. Ends often have ruler to allow depth assessment.

Varieties: Rubber, metal, or plastic handles. Various lengths of awl.

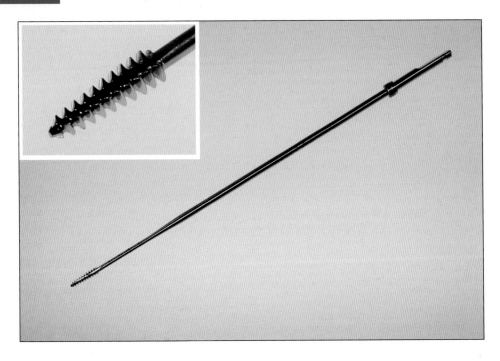

Pedicle Tap

Alternative Name: Tap

Category: Spine fusion instrumentation

Purposes: Used to place the initial bony threads to lay the foundation for screw trajectories.

Varieties: Many variables depending on manufacturer.

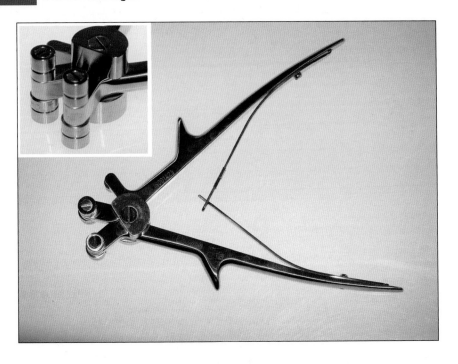

Rod Bender

Alternative Name: Bender

Category: Spine fusion instrumentation

Purposes: Allows customized bending of rods.

Varieties: Various sizes of instrument to accommodate different sizes of rods.

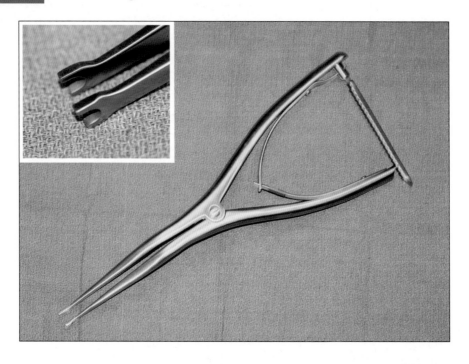

Rod Distractor

Alternative Name: Distractor

Category: Spine fusion instrumentation

Purposes: Allows distraction of vertebral segments by seating the instrument between the screw heads. The instrument then pushes them outward.

Varieties: Various lengths.

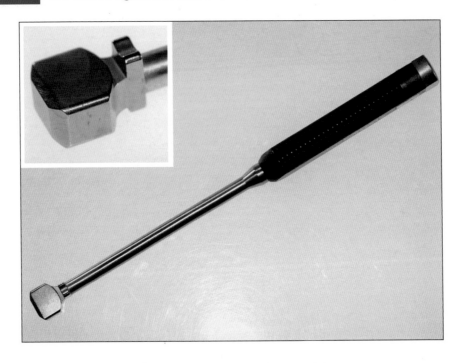

Spine Block Filler

Alternative Name: Trial

Category: Spine fusion instrumentation

Purposes: Allows assessment of desired disc interspace graft size.

Varieties: Multiple heights, widths, and angles of trial.

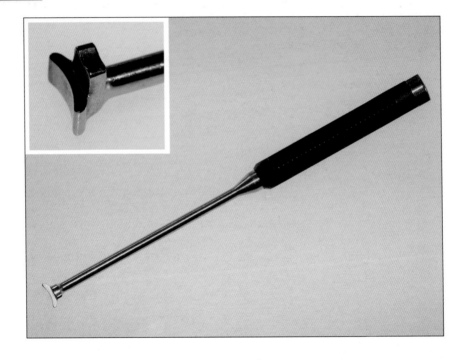

Spine Graft Impactor

Alternative Names: Graft impactor, impactor, graft tamp, tamp

Category: Spine fusion instrumentation

Purposes: Impaction of bone graft or other structure, e.g., cage, into place. Used with a mallet.

Varieties: Various lengths. Smooth or sharp end. Metal, plastic, or wood handles.

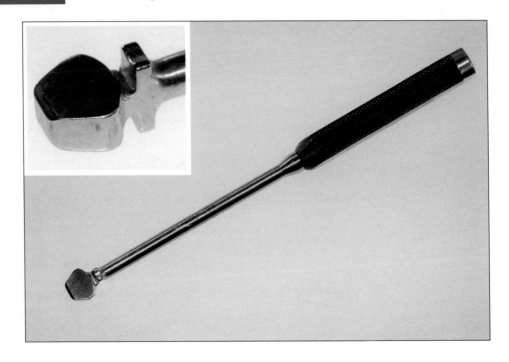

Spine Graft Implant Trial

Alternative Name: Trial

Category: Spine fusion instrumentation

Purposes: Allows assessment of desired disc interspace graft size.

Varieties: Multiple heights, widths, and angles of trial.

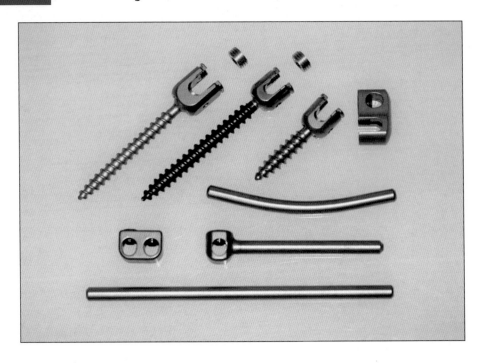

Spine Instrumentation

Alternative Names: Screws called by measurement, rods by length, and other items by name

Category: Spine fusion instrumentation

Purposes: Instrumentation designed to provide stability of the spine during fusion procedure. Countless variations allow for infinite fusion solutions. Most common construction consists of rods connecting consecutively instrumented segments.

Varieties: Many variables depending on manufacturer.

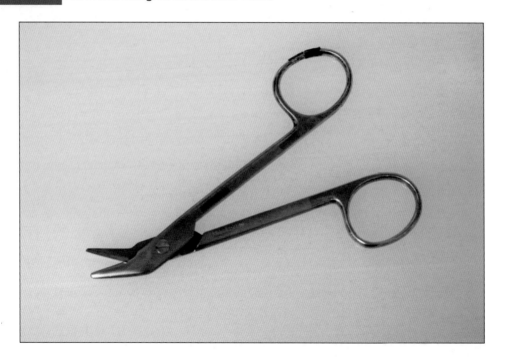

Wire Cutters

Alternative Name: None

Category: Spine fusion instrumentation

Purposes: Trimming or cutting wire, often used in spinal stabilization procedures.

Varieties: Various lengths.

Chapter 7: Transsphenoidal/Endonasal

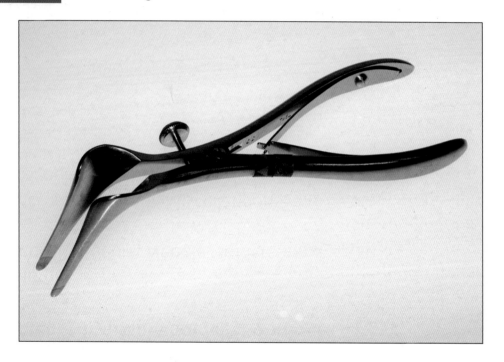

Cottle Speculum

Alternative Names: Nasal speculum, Killian speculum, nasal spreader, nare speculum

Category: Retractors

Purposes: Used for retraction of the nares to improve visualization during transsphenoidal/endo-nasal procedures. This retractor is self-retaining.

Varieties: Variable blade lengths and widths.

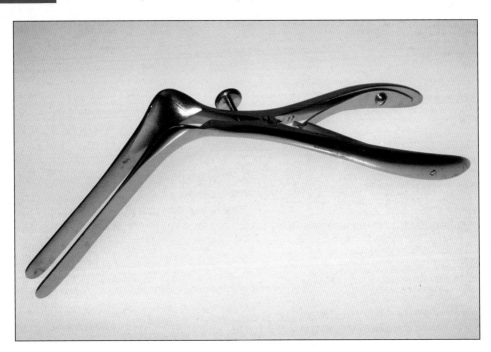

Killian Speculum

Alternative Names: Nasal speculum, Cottle speculum, nasal spreader, nare speculum

Category: Retractors

Purposes: Used for retraction of the nares to improve visualization during transsphenoidal/endonasal procedures. This retractor is self-retaining.

Varieties: Variable blade lengths and widths.

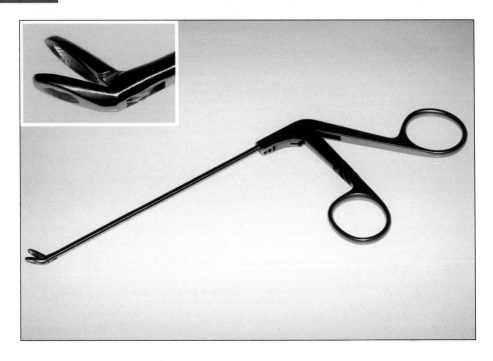

Blakesley Wilde Rhinoforce Forceps

Alternative Name: Blakesley forceps

Category: Forceps

Purposes: Endonasal/endoscopical manipulation of delicate tissues.

Varieties: Straight or angled jaws or blades.

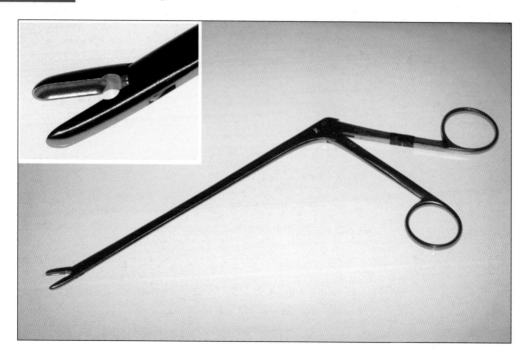

Takahashi Forceps

Alternative Names: Pituitary, tissue forceps

Category: Forceps

Purposes: Grasping and manipulating tissue during transsphenoidal/endonasal cases. Can be used for tissue grasping and biopsy samples in cranial and spinal cases.

Varieties: Straight or angled jaws. Various jaw sizes. Variable length of instrument.

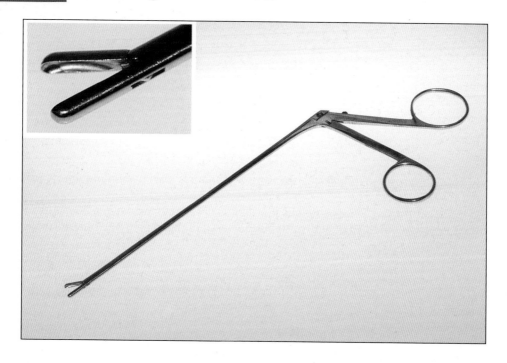

Decker Micro Rongeur

Alternative Names: Decker forceps, endoscopic Takahashi, endoscopic forceps, biopsy forceps

Category: Rongeurs

Purposes: Manipulation of delicate tissues in deep, small spaces, especially in transsphenoidal/endonasal, spinal, and deep cranial cases. The jaws allow biopsy material, cyst wall, or other soft tissue to be securely taken.

Varieties: Length and diameter of shaft. Straight, directional, or angled jaws. Variable width of jaws.

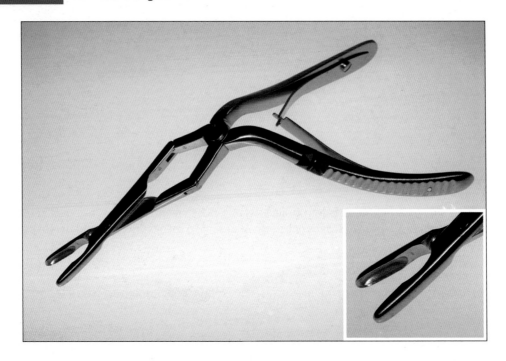

Jansen-Middleton Rongeur

Alternative Names: Angled rongeur, angled septal rongeur

Category: Rongeurs

Purposes: Angled rongeurs for transsphenoidal/endonasal cases for the removal of bony material, mainly the septum. Can be used as forceps as well.

Varieties: None.

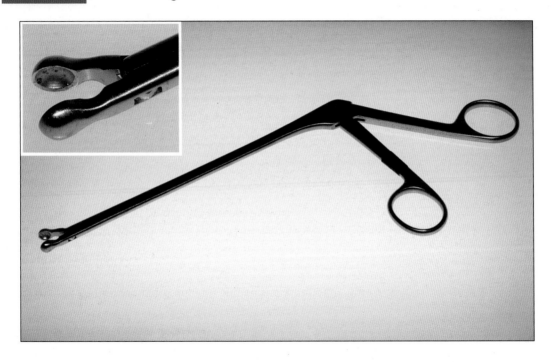

Oldberg Rongeur

Alternative Names: Bateman pituitary forceps, pituitary, tissue graspers, biopsy forceps

Category: Rongeurs

Purposes: Used for grasping and manipulating tissue during transsphenoidal/endonasal cases. Often used for tissue biopsy.

Varieties: Various cup sizes. Variable length of instrument.

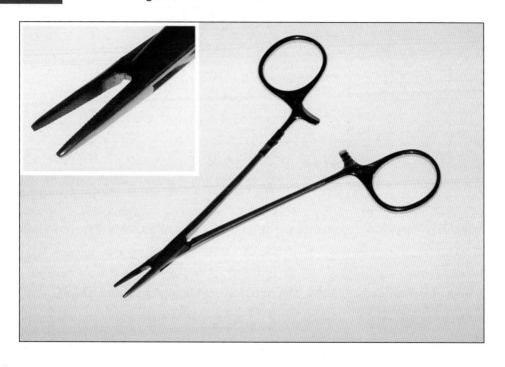

Webster Needle Holder

Alternative Names: Baumgartner needle holder, Derf needle holder, Par needle holder, pediatric needle holder, small needle holder, needle driver

Category: Needle holders

Purposes: Small needle holder with jaws that allow movement of the needle without releasing the jaws. Also used with smaller needles.

Varieties: Smooth or serrated jaws. Various lengths. Various materials.

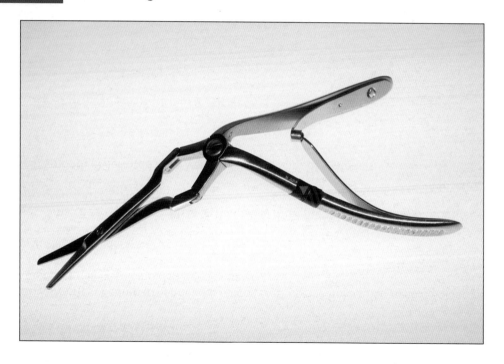

Becker Septum Scissors

Alternative Names: Septum scissors, double-action septum scissors

Category: Scissors

Purposes: Used for cutting septal tissue in transsphenoidal/endonasal procedures.

Varieties: None.

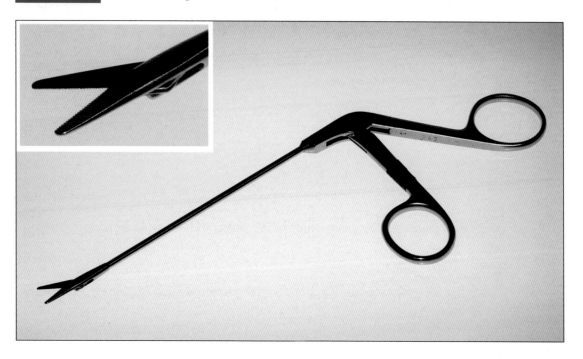

Blakesley Wilde Rhinoforce Scissors

Alternative Name: Blakesley scissors

Category: Scissors

Purposes: Endonasal/endoscopic manipulation of or cutting of delicate tissues.

Varieties: Straight or angled jaws or blades.

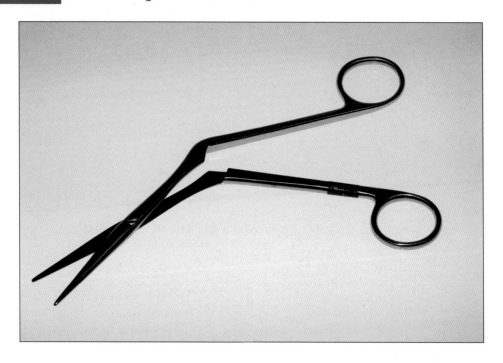

Knight Nasal Scissors

Alternative Names: Meisterhand Knight scissors, Fomon, Heymann, Cottle scissors, nasal scissors

Category: Scissors

Purposes: Used for cutting nasal mucosa and soft tissue. Most often used in transsphenoidal/endonasal cases.

Varieties: Straight or curved blades. Various lengths of blades and arms.

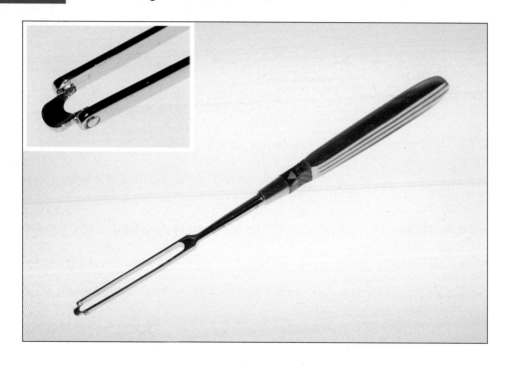

Ballenger Swivel Knife

Alternative Names: Swivel or Ballenger knife

Category: Knives

Purposes: Resection of tissue in small spaces, especially turbinae in transsphenoidal/endonasal procedures.

Varieties: Straight or bayonet.

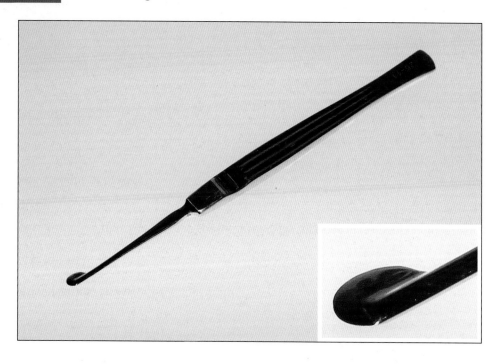

Freer Knife

Alternative Names: Pierce septal knife, septal knife

Category: Knives

Purposes: Used for cutting and dissecting tissue off and from the septum during transsphenoidal/endonasal cases. Can be used in other cases for fine dissection of delicate tissue, e.g., large cranial or spinal tumors.

Varieties: None.

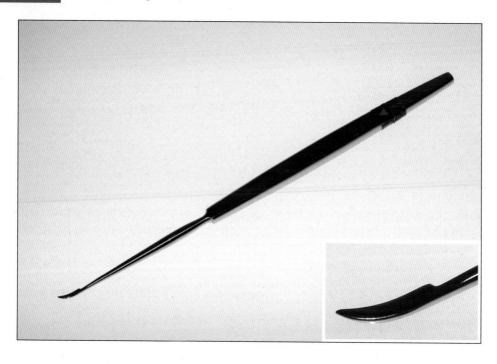

Sickle Knife

Alternative Names: House sickle, House knife, Sexton ear knife, curved knife

Category: Knives

Purposes: Cutting and dissecting tool often used in transsphenoidal/endonasal cases for creation of septal flaps. Can be used in any procedure requiring a long-handled knife for non-delicate tissue cutting and dissection.

Varieties: Reusable or disposable.

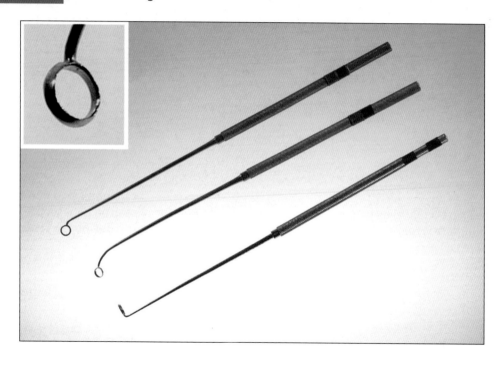

Hardy Curette

Alternative Names: Sklar curette, Rogozinski curette, cone ring curette, ring curette

Category: Dissectors

Purposes: Used to dissect and mobilize soft tissue in a confined space, e.g., transsphenoidal/endonasal or large craniospinal tumors. The edges of the ring allow a continued orthogonal force to be applied and the subsequent removal of tissue without obstruction from the previously removed tissue.

Varieties: Straight, curved, or angled shafts. Bayonet or straight handles. Various lengths of shaft.

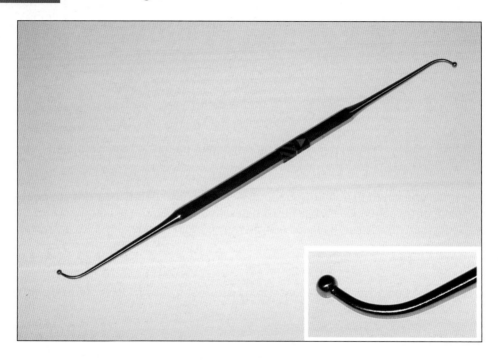

Maxillary Ostium Seeker

Alternative Names: Ostium probe, ostium seeker

Category: Dissectors

Purposes: Double-ended ball tip probe used to find the ostium in transsphenoidal/endonasal cases.

Varieties: Single- or double-ended.

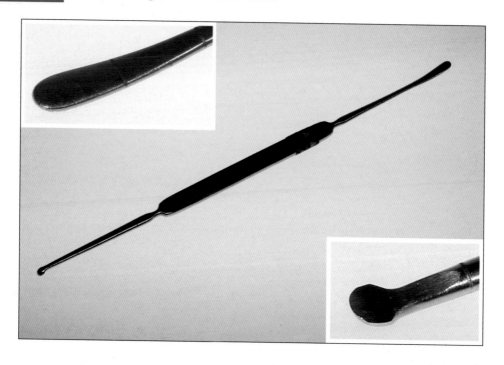

Cottle Elevator

Alternative Names: Septal elevator, mucosa elevator

Category: Elevators

Purposes: Double-ended instrument with a sharp, flat end and the other with a teardrop shape, allowing the dissection of delicate soft tissue off, most commonly, the septum. However, this elevator can be used to separate the dura, ligament, or other soft tissue from bone.

Varieties: None.

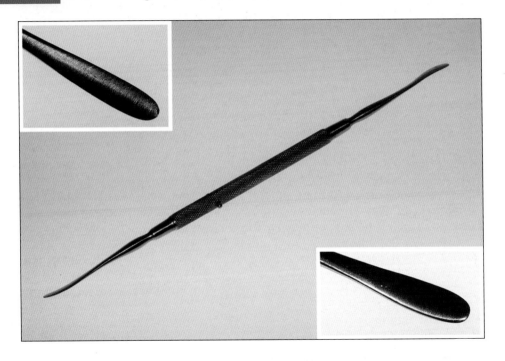

Freer Elevator

Alternative Names: Cottle elevator, Pierce elevator, submucosal elevator

Category: Elevators

Purposes: Multipurpose tool used to separate soft tissue from bone, e.g., nasal septum, skull base, dura, etc. to dissect vascular plaque in endarterectomies; and even as a protection device when drilling or placing bone wax for hemostasis in narrow spaces.

Varieties: Single- or double-ended. Sharp or blunt blades.

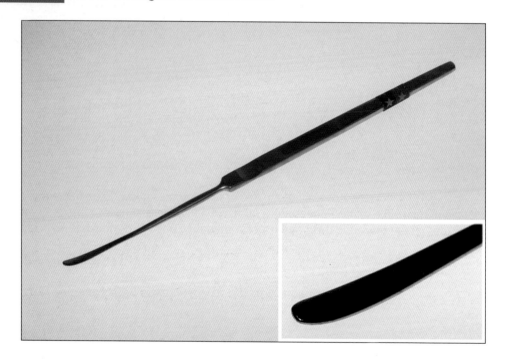

Halle Elevator

Alternative Names: Elevator, tissue elevator, septal elevator (incorrect), Penfield 4 (incorrect)

Category: Elevators

Purposes: Multipurpose tool used in separating soft tissue from bone, e.g., nasal septum, skull base, dura, etc., and even as a protection device when drilling or placing bone wax for hemostasis in narrow spaces.

Varieties: None.

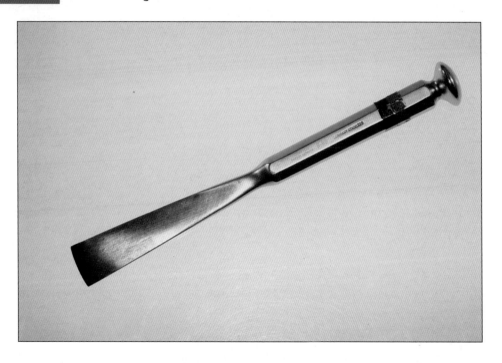

Chisel

Alternative Names: Hibbs chisel, Hoke chisel, osteotome

Category: Miscellaneous

Purposes: Used for any modification or sculpting of bone. Selected cranial or spinal cuts, bone graft harvest, and/or molding. Should be used with a mallet.

Varieties: The cutting end can be straight or curved. The length of the shaft and width of the cutting blade come in many combinations. The more common are 15 to 25 cm in length and 4 to 25 mm in width.

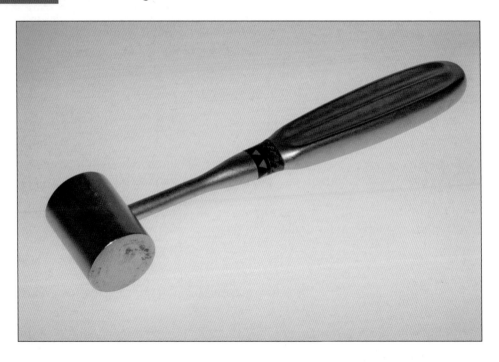

Cottle Mallet

Alternative Names: Mallet, hammer

Category: Miscellaneous

Purposes: Used for application of force, usually on another instrument, e.g., osteotome, bone graft impactor, chisel, etc.

Varieties: Variable weights. Variable material for mallet head and handle.

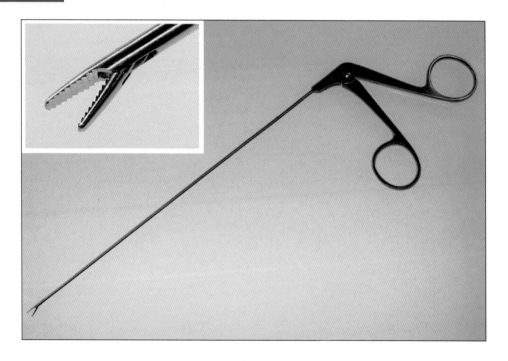

Endodscopic Grasping Forceps

Alternative Names: Endo forceps, Takahashis

Category: Forceps

Purposes: Grasping and holding forceps designed for endoscopic use.

Varieties: Straight or angled jaws. Variable width of jaws. Sharp or smooth jaws.

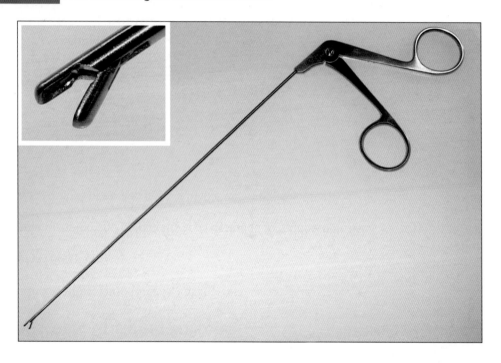

Endoscopic Biopsy Forceps

Alternative Names: Endoscopic Takahashi, endoscopic forceps, biopsy forceps

Category: Forceps

Purposes: Used for endoscopically manipulating delicate tissues. The cups allow biopsy material or cyst wall material to be securely taken, especially in endoscopic ventricular or pediatric cases.

Varieties: Length and diameter of shaft. Straight or angled jaws.

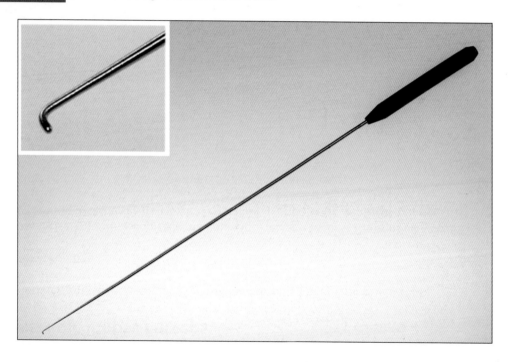

Endoscopic Long Nerve Hook

Alternative Names: Nerve hook, long Dandy hook

Category: Dissectors

Purposes: Exploring, probing, and dissecting fine delicate soft tissue and nerves, often used to inspect underneath and within structures. The rounded handle allows a rolling, twisting action to sweep tissue away or to work the instrument between tissue planes.

Varieties: Length and angle of tip. Length of shaft.

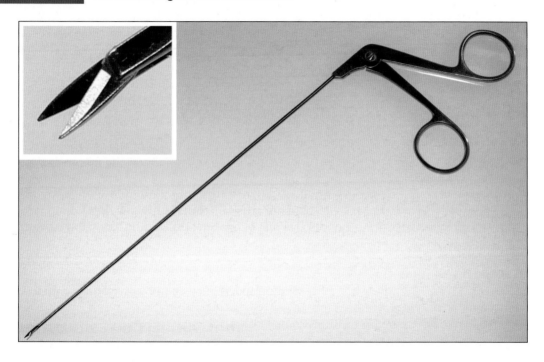

Endoscopic Scissors

Alternative Names: Micro scissors, endoscopic scissors

Category: Scissors

Purposes: Endoscopic scissors used for cutting and dissecting delicate soft tissue.

Varieties: Straight, curved, or angled blades. Various lengths of arms.

Appendix

Neurosurgical Instrument Distributors, Suppliers, and Manufacturers

Adeor (adeor.com)

Aesculap (aesculapinc.com)

Anspach (anspach.com)

ASSI (accuratesurgical.com)

Biomet (biomet.com)

Codman and Shurtleff (depuy.com)

DePuy (depuy.com)

Electro Surgical Instrument Company (electrosurgicalinstrument.com)

Fehling Surgical Instruments Inc (fehlingsurgical.com)

GerMedUSA Inc (germedusa.com)

Globus Medical (globusmedical.com)

HNM Medical (hnmmedical.com)

Integra Life Sciences (integralife.com)

Jarit (integralife.com/jarit)

Karl Storz (karlstorz.de)

Leica Microsystems (leica-microsystems.com)

Life Instruments (lifeinstruments.com)

Lorenz Surgical (lorenzsurgical.com)

Medicon Instrumente (medicon.de)

Medtronic (medtronic.com)

Millenium Surgical Corp (milleniumsurgical.com)

Miltex (medicalresources.com)

Mizuho (mizuho.com)

NuVasive (nuvasive.com)

Roboz (roboz.com)

Ruggles Instrument Inc (integralife.com)

Scanlan International (scanlaninternational.com)

Sklar Instruments (sklarcorp.com)

Stealth Surgical (stealthsurgical.com)

Stryker (stryker.com)

Surgical Tools Inc (surgicaltools.com)

Synthes (synthes.com)

Ulrich Medical USA (ulrichmedicalusa.com)

Whittemore Enterprises (wemed1.com)

World Federation for Neurosurgical Societies (wfns.org)

Zeiss (zeiss.com)